LUPUS

Real Life Patients Talk

Marisa Zeppieri-Caruana

Lupus: Real Life, Real Patients, Real Talk

ISBN-13: 978-0-615-80877-2

ISBN-10: 0615808778

A THOUGHTS & LETTERS
PRESS
PUBLICATION

A DIVISION OF THOUGHTS &
LETTERS, INC.

NEW YORK

Lupus: Real Life, Real Patients, Real Talk

Marisa Zeppieri-Caruana

Featuring

Lupus Foundation of America Southeast Florida Chapter CEO, Amy Kelly-Yalden,

and

Magdalena Cadet, MD, FACR, Director of Rheumatology at New York Presbyterian Healthcare System/New York Hospital Queens and Assistant Professor of Clinical Medicine/Weill Cornell Medical College

More information can be found at

www.LupusSurvivalGuide.com

This book is dedicated to the women who raised me –

My grandmother, Rose, who was my tower of strength and shared her endless love of books with me.

My mother, Patricia, whose unconditional love and tender spirit sustains me.

A portion of proceeds from this book will be donated to the Lupus Foundation of America, Southeast Florida Chapter

TABLE OF CONTENTS

Foreword 1

Why I Wrote This Book 3

Share Your Story 7

CHAPTER 1 9

Perspective Highlight · A Physician's Perspective

CHAPTER 2 15

The Story of Tanique Rose

CHAPTER 3 27

The Story of Naomi Jeanty

CHAPTER 4 39

The Story of Wendy D. Phillips

CHAPTER 5 55

The Story of Damian Velez

CHAPTER 6 65

The Story of Kathleen Walker

CHAPTER 7...77

The Story of Laurie Renfro

CHAPTER 8...87

Perspective Highlight: A Mother's Point of View

CHAPTER 9...91

The Story of Linda Bernal Apgar

CHAPTER 10.. 101

The Story of Nicole H. Francis

CHAPTER 11.. 109

The Story of PJ Nunn

CHAPTER 12.. 121

The Story of Kia Paynes-Gentry

CHAPTER 13.. 127

The Story of Kim Green

CHAPTER 14.. 135

The Story of Patty Guidice

CHAPTER 15.. 143

Perspective Highlight · A Sister's Perspective

CHAPTER 16.. 149

The Story of Elijah Julian Samaroo

CHAPTER 17.. 159

The Story of Jody Ortiz

CHAPTER 18.. 167

The Story of Jessica Goldman Foung

CHAPTER 19.. 179

The Story of Jonathan A. Ramirez

CHAPTER 20.. 191

The Story of Marisa Zeppieri-Caruana

CHAPTER 21.. 207

Perspective Highlight – A Best Friend's Perspective

CHAPTER 22.. 211

Perspective Highlight – A Husband's Perspective

About the Author.. 219

Acknowledgements.. 221

In Memory Of… 227

Foreword

My sister, Erin, died from complications of lupus in 2009 when she was just 34 years old. Following her death, I read her journal. Although we were the best of friends, I never could have imagined how alone and isolated she felt living with lupus since the age of 19. Now I can. As the President and CEO of the Lupus Foundation of America's Southeast Florida Chapter (LFA) since 2010, I now know that most individuals living with lupus feel the same way. This disease is cruel and mysterious. There is little to no awareness and a lack of empathy among the general population. There is no cure and there has only been one treatment option in over 52 years.

I have had the pleasure to meet many people living with this disease over the years. One in particular, Marisa Zeppieri-Caruana, also a board member of the LFA, has never ceased to amaze me with her drive and desire to tell the story of this disease. Marisa's story in itself will leave you in awe of this young woman's determination in the midst of this disease attacking her body and changing her life and her dreams completely. Instead of feeling sorry for herself, Marisa made new dreams and reached out to others whose lives have been turned upside down by lupus. She shared her story and in turn, they shared theirs.

This book is the culmination of those heartfelt and honest exchanges.

Whether you are living with lupus, love someone with lupus, lost someone to lupus, are looking to educate yourself about this disease, or simply desire to read stories of individuals who will make you view your own life differently, this book is for you. It will make you cry. It will make you smile. It will make you angry. It will make you cheer for the triumphs. It will inspire you to find the blessings in life's struggles.

This book will also ensure that the five million plus people living with lupus in this world no longer have to feel alone. Although lupus affects every single person's body in different ways, one thing is a constant, it is easier to live with this disease knowing that there is a community of others who know its' cruel and mysterious effects, have a will to make the best of their situation, and even find blessings on their journey.

Heartfelt thanks to Marisa and every individual who shared their stories and their hearts in this wonderful book. I only wish it had been published a few years earlier.

Amy Kelly-Yalden
President and CEO
Lupus Foundation of America Southeast Florida Chapter
www.lupusfl.org

Why I Wrote This Book

On April 22, 2001, my life was forever changed. On that day, I was run over by a speeding pick-up truck, driven by a drunk driver, while I walked to my car. This would be the first time I almost lost my life. The physical trauma caused by the accident ignited a series of events over the next few weeks that ultimately led to a diagnosis of Systemic Lupus at the age of 23. My doctors believed that I likely had the disease brewing within me for some time (based on my prior health history), but the accident brought my body to such a weakened state, the disease came out in full force.

While being diagnosed with any illness is frightening, what truly scared me at the time was the mystery surrounding the disease. Twelve years ago, not many people spoke about Lupus or were familiar with the term, let alone knew what the disease involved. It was a time filled with mixed emotions, ranging from sadness, fear, anxiety and denial. Luckily, a few months after my diagnosis, I met a remarkable woman named Jiwa who was my age and who also had lupus. I felt a sense of relief – I now had someone who understood what I was going through and she was kind enough to share her personal experiences with me. Forming that relationship with her was a tremendous help. She showed me that you could still live life to the fullest, despite living with a chronic disease. Our friendship made me realize how important it is to have a support system when you are dealing with an illness; it also lit a fire within me to reach out to others who are frightened, just as I once was.

During the first seven years after my diagnosis, I created a website, LupusSurvivalGuide.com, in order to share information about the disease with others. Emails from patients, family members and friends came in from around the world inquiring about the disease. Eventually, I decided to have a section on the website that shared personal stories. Although only a few people at the time were willing to share their most intimate experiences with the disease, those stories affected others in a way I could have never imagined. The letters I read would literally cause me to weep tears of sadness and joy. Men and women of all ages were so thankful to read stories they could relate to, meet people they could reach out to, and most of all, have hope they could hold on to.

Over time, I wanted to take LupusSurvivalGuide.com to the next level and attempted to form a 501-c3. Unfortunately, my own health problems were too severe at the time. Between mini-strokes, heart problems, blood clots, major infections and periods of being wheelchair or bed bound, I had to come up with another way that I could help others with lupus. I began volunteering, when my health allowed, for the Lupus Foundation of America,

Southeast Florida Chapter. Eventually, I became a support group leader and after a few years, I was invited to serve on their Board of Directors. During this time, I also began my career as a freelance journalist. Writing has opened up a world and life for me that I could never have imagined. I feel as though God has handed me the perfect career – I can still be productive, I can work from bed (or the hospital) if necessary, I love what I do, and best of all, I have a platform that can reach millions of people. So, what do I want to do with this platform? Reach out to the lupus community and talk about lupus, of course!

Two years ago, God put it on my heart to share the stories of the men and women who live every day with this disease. I envisioned a book that focused on how an individual can thrive and live the life they are meant to live, even though they are fighting for their life every day. And so, I began my quest for Lupus "thrivers" who were willing to share a glimpse into their daily lives. I thought about the type of book I could have benefited from when I was first diagnosed. I considered the questions that ran through my mind the most during those first two years, and I modeled this book from those questions; not medical information questions, but rather questions related to daily life that deal with the emotional, psychological and spiritual aspects of the disease. Although I believe this book can offer hope and inspiration to all Lupus patients in some way, I specifically dedicate it to those who are newly diagnosed and want raw truths about living each day with this disease.

I believe you hold a special and unique book in your hands.

It contains unedited and personal experiences from some of the most incredible men and women I have ever had the pleasure of interviewing. As I read each story, I was overcome with emotion. Many times, I had to walk away from the computer. Lupus is a vicious disease, but the men and women who openly share their stories in this book show you the disease has not taken away their will to live and their hope. Although the book itself went through an editing process, I left each individual's answers exactly as they were given to me. At first, I considered turning each interview into a story, but later realized their answers were so touching and personal, they had more of an impact when left in a "Question & Answer" format.

Lupus is a mysterious, frightening and callous disease. Although living with the disease is a daily struggle, there is hope. The following men and women are proof. I hope this collection of stories changes your life and inspires you to live, despite a daunting medical diagnosis. I believe inspiration brings forth motivation, and when you combine those two, you have the power to do something extraordinary with your life.

Marisa Zeppieri-Caruana
Author and Board Member, LFA Southeast Florida

Share Your Story

I would like to invite you to share your story for the second edition of this book. Please send your contact information and a brief introduction to MarisaZeppieri@gmail.com.

I would also love to hear your reactions to the stories and perspectives shared in this book. Please feel free to email me about your favorite story or which stories impacted you the most.

I hope you enjoy reading this book as much as I have enjoyed compiling the interviews and writing it.

Marisa Zeppieri-Caruana

CHAPTER 1

Perspective Highlight - A Physician's Perspective

By Magdalena Cadet, MD, FACR
Director of Rheumatology
New York Presbyterian Healthcare System/New York
Hospital Queens
Assistant Professor of Clinical Medicine/Weill Cornell
Medical College
Board Certified in Internal Medicine and Rheumatology

I can remember the first time I heard the words "Systemic Lupus Erythematosus" (SLE).

I was in my second year of medical school and a friend had complained of several months of joint pain and swelling, extreme fatigue, weight loss, and mild hair loss. Then, one day she told me she had been diagnosed with lupus. At that point in medical school, I barely knew the details of this disease. From lectures, I recalled that it was considered to be a type of autoimmune disease. Autoimmune diseases are illnesses that occur when the body's tissues are attacked by its own immune system. Patients with autoimmune diseases produce proteins or antibodies in their blood that target tissues within their own body rather than foreign infectious agents like viruses and bacteria, resulting in inflammation. At the time, I believed that arthritis associated with autoimmune diseases only affected older patients and only involved the joints. I later learned this was a myth. In my limited experience, I thought of arthritis as many other people did, as tennis or golfer's elbow, Achilles tendonitis, or bursitis. This was another myth.

How could my young friend have arthritis, let alone an autoimmune disease?

I could tell my friend was also in disbelief about her diagnosis. Moreover, she was given a therapeutic regimen that consisted of high dose steroids and other immunosuppressive agents. She did not want to take these medicines because they made her face look fat and she felt bloated and hungry all the time. I could relate to her insecurities, because I too was a girl in my mid-twenties at the time. She admitted to me that she would skip her doses of medications on some days. Back then, I was unaware that skipping a few doses of medications could make such a great difference in how well the disease was controlled.

She never fully understood the extent of her disease. For example, she was unaware of the association of early heart disease, lung disease, or kidney damage that can occur with SLE if early and aggressive treatment is not taken to control disease activity. I also did not understand how serious this disease could be, or I would have tried harder to persuade her to follow up with doctors and take her medications regularly. Several months after her diagnosis, I received the tragic and surprising news that she had passed away from complications of the disease. I learned that she had stopped taking the medications in the last few weeks before her death because she felt that her disease was localized to her joints and felt she could cope with the joint pain. She did not know the connection between her arthritis and her other organs, particularly her heart, lungs, kidneys, brain, and gastrointestinal tract.

After medical school, I made the decision to pursue my interest in the field of rheumatology, the specialty that focuses on the diagnosis and treatment of diseases of joints, muscles, and bone that exhibit systemic inflammation. I knew that, as a young physician, I could use the poignant medical school experience to relate to the young and middle-aged women who are often the targets of this disease. After my residency at Yale New Haven Hospital, I pursued my training in rheumatology at NYU/Hospital for Joint Diseases in NYC. During my fellowship, I was given the opportunity to work in a special lupus clinic every week, where I encountered amazing women living with this disease.

My patients came from several ethnic and socio-economic backgrounds. I marveled at how these women lived their daily lives, carrying out their roles as mothers, daughters, sisters, students, employers/employees, professionals and caretakers while battling this disease, which could affect any organ system at any time. These women accomplished so much, all while taking drugs · powerful immunosuppressants · such as steroids or chemotherapy agents like cyclophosphamide (Cytoxan). While these medications could help to halt the progression of the disease, they also brought about burdensome side effects, such as weight gain, bone loss, hair loss, acne, bone marrow suppression, and severe fatigue.

I also noticed that although any race could be affected, I mostly saw minority populations living with lupus, especially African Americans, Afro-Caribbean, Hispanics, and Asian females. I was happy to discover that, as an African American/Haitian female physician, I helped them feel more comfortable coming to me for aid. I explained to these women the complex factors —which included environmental, hormonal, and genetic influences—that could affect the immune system and contribute to the development of the disease. It was also important to sit down and discuss the co-morbidities associated with lupus, such as, accelerated and premature cardiovascular disease (atherosclerosis); the development of early diabetes from steroid use; premature bone loss or osteoporosis; kidney failure; and premature ovarian failure from the immunosuppressive therapies. I knew that I would continue to meet inspiring people living with SLE as I continued to practice rheumatology.

Although I have seen the ugly side of this disease, I have also witnessed the success stories.

About two years ago, I was invited to a cosmetic workshop at Bloomingdales in NYC and Bobbi Brown was the surprise guest. I was so elated to get some tips on how to be a glamour girl. After the workshop, women were paired off with a Bobbi Brown makeup artist. I was immediately taken to a woman (named Faith) who appeared to be so energetic, vibrant, and not to mention, very pretty. We instantly connected as we started to chatter. Sometime in the middle of the conversation, I told her what I did for a living. When I told her that I was a rheumatologist, her eyes widened with amazement and told me that she has been living with SLE for many years. We proceeded to talk for the next hour about how she grew up coping with the disease and how she refused to let this disease control her life. She continued to tell me how she was diagnosed at age eighteen while she was a freshman in college. She had complaints of joint pain and chest pain from inflammation around her heart. Her disease was complicated by kidney failure requiring weekly dialysis and eventually two kidney transplants. She developed a blood clot in her leg after the first transplant and her first transplanted kidney was removed within hours after the initial surgical procedure. She told me at the time that she would be celebrating her two-year anniversary of her successful second kidney transplant in December 2010. She also reported being treated with several years of steroids, chemotherapy (cyclophosphamide) and other agents. She is now on a regimen of low dose steroids and anti-rejection medications. It was great to see this amazing forty year old, married professional in one of the best cosmetic companies of the world stand before me after enduring two kidney transplants. At the end of my makeover, we exchanged our contact information and I promised her that I would write about her. Meeting Faith was a sign that with an early diagnosis, aggressive treatment, a healthy lifestyle, a supportive physician, social network, and a positive outlook on life, this disease can be controlled.

I see women on a daily basis in my practice who live with the strength and courage to wake up every day and fight this disease by keeping their disease activity in remission with the help of caring physicians, potent medications and healthy lifestyle modifications. Snoop Dog's daughter was recently seen on the View in 2010 opening up about her battle with juvenile SLE. Every day when I go to work, I keep the faces of the girls and women that I have treated and cared for in my mind and in my heart. When I think of them, I know that I have chosen the right vocation. These females inspire me to increase awareness about the clinical symptoms, diagnostic evaluation, complications like atherosclerosis and treatment associated with this disease. Please take the time out to read this story and share with any male or female that may have symptoms suspicious for SLE. That person should immediately be referred to a rheumatologist.

I wish my friend from medical school knew what I know today about this disease. I wish she could have met Faith and realized that living a long, happy and productive life with Systemic Lupus Erythematosus is possible

.

CHAPTER 2

The Story of Tanique Rose

Miami, Florida
24 years of age
Administrative Assistant

Q: Tanique, how you were diagnosed with lupus? What was happening in your life during that period, what age were you, and what type of symptoms were you experiencing?

A: I was diagnosed at the young age of 21. As a hardworking student in college, taking four critical courses to finish my degree, I never thought twice about my health. Living my life with friends, enjoying late nights, studying all day and into the night, I never thought about the stress I caused on my body.

One day I felt a horrible pain shoot through my joints as I waited in my car before class · I remember this vividly as it was the first time I felt anything like this. Sitting in my car studying before class was something I did regularly. I did not understand what I did differently this time to deserve the crippling pain I felt as I sat trying to pull myself together. I called my mother to ask questions about the pain because I figured she might have an idea. She quickly told me to come home and see my doctor. Instead, I decided to push through the pain that day and other days until the semester was over.

In late December of that year, 2009, days before New Year's Eve, I tested positive for lupus. My doctor advised me to find a rheumatologist and luckily, I found an incredible doctor. I did my research and found out I had more symptoms of lupus than I had ever paid attention to.

Q: How would you describe your initial reaction to the diagnosis? Were you somewhat expecting it or did it come as a shock to you?

A: I was shocked! My family was also shocked and my husband, who was my fiancée at the time, took it hard. I am and will always be a hardworking, self-driven woman, but when I got the news, I knew I had to be stronger for my family to feel secure with the situation. For almost the first two years, the only people that knew were my parents and my husband. I eventually told my close circle of friends in 2010; I was afraid and embarrassed to discuss what I was going through. I finally told my sisters in 2011. Other family and friends found out when I created an event page on Facebook for the Walk for Lupus Now 2012 event and invited them to participate. Although this diagnosis was something I never expected to happen to me, I am adjusting day by day.

Q: How does your initial reaction to the diagnosis differ from your outlook on life today?

A: Today, I have become more educated about lupus (SLE). I have embraced it as something that was added to my life. I have to stay strong because that is the type of person I was raised to be. If I let this disease control my life, I will not have a life. My support system is limitless. My rheumatologist is amazing with the advice she provides about how to live healthy. I do fear the reality of being caught off guard again by a flare-up, possibly worse than I have ever experienced. Joint pain, serious fatigue, and other symptoms affect my daily life, but I refuse to take medications that will alter my natural health.

Q: What are some tangible lessons that you would like to share with a newly diagnosed person or someone who is struggling with the disease?

A: As a lupus patient, knowing my particular symptoms was very important. Educating yourself can help develop a better lifestyle. When I realized fatigue was an issue for me, I minimized my time in the sun and now take extra time to rest and rejuvenate my body. There was a time in my life when sleep was not a priority and that is what pushed my body over the edge. Eating healthy has been a major part of my life since the day I was diagnosed. I revamped my life and my diet by learning which fruits and vegetables give me certain nutrients. Educating my friends so they could understand that resting is essential to my health was a major part of my lupus experience. If you are a student in college, it is okay to take fewer classes. You have to keep stress at a minimum. Stress can ruin a perfectly good day for people with lupus. Stress levels have to be maintained because it is the cause of many flare-ups. As far as my occupation is concerned, my supportive family unit allows me to work part-time because full-time work has not been an option for me at this point (due to the stress and pressure it puts on my body.) When I am sick, I undoubtedly pull back and take time for myself. In addition, exercise has been a great way to maintain lupus, as well as taking away the pressure of daily life.

Q: What has changed in your life because of the disease? Did you switch majors in college, perhaps quit your job and started a completely unrelated occupation, change your plans regarding having children, move to a different location, etc.?

A: In college, I pushed myself to the finish line to receive my Bachelor's degree. I would like to start graduate school, but it is still just an idea because of my experience with school being a major stressor in the past. Before I was diagnosed with lupus, I had a five-year plan. After I graduated from college, I would enter graduate school immediately after to maintain consistency. That plan has changed and morphed into a life-changing, inconsistent day-by-day plan. When I first moved back to Miami after college with my husband, I put my health aside to give everything I had to find a career. I applied to a different job every day. The stress of not getting called back and being rejected started to become an issue for my health. I had to recuperate from allowing my illness to become an issue. Now I take things steady and slow. I had to learn my life is no longer a game to be played with. I could not accomplish anything by jumping in headfirst regarding major decisions. Everything I do consists of planning first because of lupus.

Recently, at the beginning of 2012, my doctors told me I would have to plan my pregnancy because I am considered a high risk. That was the most devastating news I received through this whole experience – the thought of being married and not having children. My chances of having a healthy pregnancy are in the hands of doctors. My husband and I are considering our options, but have not given up on the idea of starting a family. Now we focus more on each other and enjoying our lives together until that moment we have to decide if children are in our best interest.

Q: What have you learned about yourself and your character through the lupus diagnosis? Has it made you stronger, more aware of taking care of yourself, or more compassionate?

A: Lupus has opened my eyes to believe I can live healthier through life changes. I have become more aware of my body and the impact of the disease. I have gained a new respect for my husband because he still married me after finding out about the disease and knowing the risks. Self-respect and encouragement have become the most important things in my life. You have to respect your body and encourage yourself to be better and stronger every day. Opening up about my illness to the world has given me strength to encourage others and help any way I can to bring awareness to the forefront of society. This disease has proven that my strength is beyond what the human eye can see.

Q: Do you consider yourself a fighter? What are some of the major hurdles you have had to deal with in terms of the disease? Think back to a moment you were very ill · how did you get to where you are now?

A: I consider myself a fighter because those moments when I feel life dealt me a horrible hand, I am able to pick myself up, focus on the positive, and move forward. The major hurdles I have had to deal with, in terms of lupus, have to be the fatigue and joint pain. The pain and stiffness I have experienced has caused me to miss some important events in my life. Birthday celebrations have been missed, school days, and spending time with friends. Some of those moments, I wish I could get back but I cannot. Now I am stronger because of what I have experienced. I am able to tell family and friends what I am experiencing instead of hiding it. In the past when I became sick, no one knew where I was or what I was going through. I had become so good at hiding my disease. Today I am open and honest about everything I am going through with lupus.

Q: Tanique, tell me about your support system.

A: My support system consists of my husband, father, mother and sisters. They love me unconditionally. Before my diagnosis, they knew me as the always helpful, strong-willed and determined sister, daughter and fiancé. Now in their eyes, I am still the same, but I have an "added incentive" – that is what I like to call it. My husband is a hardworking, loving man and so supportive of every decision I make. He is my main line to staying healthy and secure with myself. Even days when I feel horrible, he is right by my side telling me to rest and stop for a while. I have always been the type of person to work myself until I burn out, but he keeps me balanced. My sisters keep me motivated to do more with my life. They are younger, so I am always determined to be their role model. My father is the most loving, caring and strongest father any daughter could ever ask for. He knows what I need before I say anything and is always willing to help even when I try to deny his assistance.

Q: What would you tell a newly diagnosed person regarding the importance of having a support system?

A: I would tell them that their support system is everything. Having family and friends to motivate you when you feel like giving up is so important. Having love and affection around you when you are at your worst is crucial. When I talk to newly diagnosed lupus patients, I always tell them to open up and allow their family to support them. Let them know when you cannot make it to work. Allow them to be there when your body seems like it has had enough. Keeping the disease a secret only adds to the stress because you are holding it from people that mean a lot to you and care about you.

Q: Describe the positives in life even after a lupus diagnosis. What is your perspective on how you can lead a productive life even with the disease?

A: Living a life with lupus is not the end of your life. I can still live a productive life by knowing my limitations, but still doing the same activities I enjoy. I take trips with my husband, hang out with friends, play video games, play basketball with my sisters, and I am applying to school to continue my education. My workload will not be as big as it used to be, but I am determined to be a better me every day of my life. For instance, even though I am not as disciplined with exercise, when I can exercise, I notice a difference in the way I feel. Therefore, I exercise because it is something that makes me feel better inside and out. Even though I am working part-time, that is just the beginning of my journey.

"Never let something you can't change take control of your life." This is the motto I live by. My happiness means the world to me. Life is too short to dwell on things you cannot change; you have to learn to live with it by any means necessary.

Q: How does faith play a role in your disease? What are your beliefs and how have they helped you get through not only the difficult diagnosis, but also everyday hiccups that occur with lupus?

A: My faith in God has played a huge role in dealing with lupus. My family prays for me all the time and I pray for a better life, health and strength on a daily basis. Believing in God played a major role in my decisions with medication. I believe God is the ultimate healer. My fear of having children has gotten better through spiritual guidance and prayer as well. Having faith in God helps me get through my toughest moments with the disease. I grew up on prayer and attended church with my grandparents. They always told me if I could not handle a burden, turn to God because He can definitely handle my problems. I put my trust and my life in the hands of the ultimate healer.

Q: What role has nutrition, healthy living and exercise played in your life? Do you exercise or follow any specific eating habits? And, have you ever consulted with a nutritionist?

A: I believe nutrition is very important when living with lupus. Exercise and diet restore your health and strength. I started juicing to assure myself of the nutrients I need for energy on a daily basis. I take vitamins instead of medication to reassure my body is getting the natural nutrients it needs as well. Exercise is something I am still working on, but when I do workout, I feel so much better. I started taking Yoga and it is an amazing way to meditate and get the exercise you need. When I was in college, I used to eat on an irregular basis, and when I did eat, I was not choosing healthy meals; most of the time I ate junk food or whatever I could get my hands on while studying. When I was diagnosed, I asked my husband for help because he was a personal trainer before he took on his career. With him, I had all the resources I needed to start a healthy life.

Q: How would you finish the following sentence?

Even with lupus, my life is all I have dreamed of because...

A: Even with lupus, my life is still brighter than I could ever have imagined because my family and friends are still by my side, showing me love and care. The strength that I have now with lupus is unmatched with the strength I possessed in the past because I am fighting to become better with a purpose.

Q: If your character, your life, your dreams, etc., could be summed up in one quote or motto, what would it be and why does it mean so much to you?

A: "Living is not just existing – it is making a difference in your life by taking chances and experiencing the many things life has to offer." This quote is self-proclaimed. I believe living is more than accepting challenges; it is more about being able to tell the story after the challenge is conquered. Life is too short to let anything deter your success and happiness. If lupus becomes something I can no longer fight, I would like to feel that I lived a life of proud memories and great experiences.

Q: Who are the most important people in your life and why?

A: My husband and my family are the most important people in my life because they allow me to be myself without treating me differently because of the disease. I have always been the type of person that does not accept pity or guilt because those are the characteristics that drain the strength God gives us to live successful, strong and self-fulfilling lives.

Q: What are your plans for the future, despite lupus, and how do you plan to achieve them?

A: To let my fears go and continue to live an improved life are the simplest plans I have. The tougher plans, such as finding a career and attending college again are also attainable because I have become a new person who puts health first. When health is first, everything else follows.

Q: What are three tangible pieces of advice that you would offer to someone struggling with the disease?

A: Educate yourself every chance you get on your particular situation, utilize resources and keep up-to-date on new developments of a possible cure. Do not let lupus control who you are as a person - embrace what life has to offer and deal with it day-by-day. Always remember that nutrition plays a major role in living a healthy and productive life; it provides the energy your body needs.

Q: Last, please finish the following sentence:
Even though I was diagnosed with lupus...

A: Even though I was diagnosed with lupus, I will not let it control who I am because I have become stronger and more motivated than ever to accomplish my dreams and goals.

CHAPTER 3

The Story of Naomi Jeanty

North Miami, Florida
33 Years of Age
Medical School Graduate, currently employed as a Clinical
Research Associate

Q: Naomi, how you were diagnosed with lupus? What was happening in your life during that period, what age were you, and what type of symptoms were you experiencing?

A: I was 32 years old when I was diagnosed with Systemic Lupus Erythematosus. My symptoms began four months prior to receiving my diagnosis, while beginning a new job position. Thank God, I had my family by my side to counsel me, transport me to the emergency room and nurse me back to great health. My symptoms began in June 2011 as bilateral wrist pain. Initially, I thought it was a reversible injury from a yoga pose I did a few days earlier or possibly carpal tunnel syndrome from excessive typing at work, or even from excessive mobile phone texting! Taking references from my medical background as a medical doctor, I had to think the worst after noticing my wrist pain not only persisted for more than a week but also progressed to digital swelling and intense pain to the point I could not make a fist. So, I thought lupus and/or rheumatoid arthritis and began to ask my parents extensive questions about our family history of any unknown autoimmune diseases (since there are so many). And, the answer was "no" - not one person my parents could have thought of had any autoimmune conditions.

I proceeded to make an appointment with an orthopedic to rule out any possible injury or sprain. The orthopedic doctor explained to me that the x-ray of both my wrists was negative. However, I still had my "medical doctor" hat on and suggested to him to add a rheumatological work up for me. I did the lab work and after a few days, I received a call from my primary care physician that some of the markers for autoimmunity were positive and she referred me to a rheumatologist. I went on to see the rheumatologist and received countless prescriptions of only Medrol 7-day dose packs. My symptoms became progressively worse, from localized wrist and finger pain and swelling to generalized joint involvement from head to toe. Name a joint, and it hurt! At that point, I had come to the realization of what I could have except I was still not given a name for it! Finally, I was told it could be mixed connective tissue disorder (MCTD), "a garbage pail of diagnoses," the rheumatologist explained.

After several more appointments and as my symptoms became worse, the doctor presented me with options to begin taking low dose chemotherapeutic medications. Day by day, I was limited to my performances at work and daily activities that almost led me to depression. I thought, "How was I able to be so independent and do simple tasks and now was relying on someone to open a bottle of water for me?" Another stressor was having a new job and having to make the first impression of being late to work or calling in due to difficulty arising from bed to start the day. It had me down for a while. What chronic condition could this be? I desired another option and was prompted to seek a second opinion from another rheumatologist in order to be properly managed with medication. I requested to see an MCTD (mixed connective tissue disease) specialist who only saw MCTD patients because initially that was my diagnosis.

Without hesitation, the specialist was willing to see me. After a thorough physical examination and reviewing my medical history, he ruled out MCTD. He re-entered the examining room after I re-robed to explain what my diagnosis was. Finally! He said, "How you presented along with the physical examination and history, I believe you have what is called SLE." At that point, I was glad something was confirmed, but anxious to start treatment because my lupus was very active at that point. He further educated me on the "do and don'ts" of lupus, and the various treatments available for lupus. I felt relieved and scared at the same time. That same day I began my treatment. It was October 14, 2011.

Q: How would you describe your initial reaction to the diagnosis? Were you somewhat expecting it or did it come as a shock to you?

A: My initial reaction was fear and relief. But, if I took anything away from the series "Lost" (Season 1: Episode 1), it was to only give in to fear for five seconds and proceed to gather the tools I needed to survive and fight the good fight of this condition. I did expect the diagnosis to be lupus, given my medical background and what I studied about it while in medical school. I was not entirely surprised. The way I handle anything difficult or challenging I face in my life is to learn and grow from it. I thought after receiving my diagnosis, how can I help others with the same illness? What can be my contribution moving forward living with this?

Q: How does your initial reaction to the diagnosis differ from your outlook on life today?

A: It does not differ at all. I look at all situations in life as an exploration to something bigger - bigger then myself - especially if it will make me a better person.

Q: What are some tangible lessons that you would like to share with a newly diagnosed person or someone who is struggling with the disease?

A: First, understand you have a new "normal" as far as life is concerned. Make the necessary adjustments to reduce stress as much as possible by taking deep breaths throughout the day. At work, I take breaks in intervals... even if it is to go to the bathroom stalls to sit and do deep breathing exercises. Other times, I incorporate walking and resting. I recently purchased a pedometer to monitor the steps I take each day to incorporate in my daily activities if I am unable to make it to the gym. Do not hesitate to ask for help when you need it. There are people out there who will help. Get involved in a support group. This will help disperse your fears or reluctance about the illness and will show that you are never alone in anything you experience in life. Plan your activities ahead of time to prepare your mind and taking necessary time to rest when needed.

Q: What has changed in your life because of the disease? Did you switch majors in college, perhaps quit your job and started a completely unrelated occupation, change your plans regarding having children, move to a different location, etc.?

A: What changed most is choosing what is best for me first. I learned to become more assertive with others and not allow things to simmer within, as I would do in the past. I learned to put my health first before satisfying others.

Q: Do you consider yourself a fighter? What are some of the major hurdles you have had to deal with in terms of the disease? Think back to a moment you were very ill · how did you get to where you are now?

A: I do consider myself a fighter. A major hurdle I have had to deal with in terms of my illness was making the decision to disclose my diagnosis to my job. The reaction I received was bittersweet. However, at the end, my co-workers came to realize that at my healthiest I am able to perform my work above the optimal level. My sickest moment was in January 2012 when I became hospitalized for about a week after experiencing two episodes of chest pain. At the time of having the chest pains, I could not help but hear the echoes from the rheumatologist who diagnosed me to never ignore chest pain, especially with lupus, as we are at higher risk of developing cardiovascular disease. So I went to the ER in the evening and was found to be sinus tachycardic (having rapid heartbeat) and anemic and the ER doctor decided to "keep" me. I asked the doctor, "What do you mean 'keep me'?" She responded "...meaning you will be admitted to the hospital for further observation."

The following morning I was transported to the nearest hospital facility. During my hospital stay, I was seen by a team of specialists to rule out the cause of my chest pain. In addition, numerous amounts of lab work were done which indicated the lupus was quite active and subsequently involved my kidneys as a result of more than three grams of protein being found in my urine over a 24-hour period. The nephrologist proceeded to order a kidney biopsy and the results came back few days after my hospital discharge. Aggressive treatment was initiated for lupus nephritis—an inflammation of the kidneys. Now I am stronger because of the faith I have in God through Christ, my Savior. It is because of Him and the prayers and tremendous support of my family and friends that helped me move along and push through this.

Q: Naomi, tell me about your support system.

A: My support system consists of my family and friends. From the beginning, my family has been the backbone in all of this. My sister would drop everything to transport me to the emergency room. My mother prepared meals, and soothed the pain I was having with naturopathic teas and massage. My father gathered information for me to read and purchase healthy foods to incorporate into my diet. My friends have been a blessing as well during my hospital stay—receiving multiple calls to see how I was feeling. I have a great support system.

Q: What would you tell a newly diagnosed person regarding the importance of having a support system?

A: Having a support system will first tell you that you are not alone with this condition. Personally, having someone to talk to with lupus not only made me feel good internally, because it is not a one-person battle, but it internalized an automatic family and friendship link that no one can break apart. My first encounter with another lupus patient was one of the most unforgettable moments as a newly diagnosed patient. I was very emotional because she immediately embraced me. To see another face with lupus, whose countenance radiated with life, expressed to me that difficult moments were outweighed with her empowerment to live joyfully and as healthy as possible. I believe having that support system through family, friends and other lupus patients is monumental in building a strong sense of well-being and achieving to getting better.

Q: Describe the positives in life even after a lupus diagnosis. What is your perspective on how you can lead a productive life even with the disease?

A: Continue to be yourself. Be the person before the diagnosis, but better. Think about some great lessons to learn beyond having this disease. This answer may not be immediately available, but with time, you will begin to see that your role in having this condition can impact someone or a population in your life. Living above it and continuing to press on can be that one major positive factor and I think it is the most important because you are proclaiming that you are above this and will continue to persevere in your life. I know there may be rough days ahead or you have already gone through those rough days, but seeing yourself and enriching yourself beyond this through accomplishing your dreams and desires in life is powerful in itself.

Q: How does faith play a role in your disease? What are your beliefs and how have they helped you get through not only the difficult diagnosis, but also everyday hiccups that occur with lupus?

A: My faith plays a very significant role in my life, period. After my diagnosis, for some reason, I never questioned "Why me?" I do not know why that never entered my mind but I just thought God chose me to have this to raise awareness of lupus and to enrich my growth in Him. Maybe it was to remember God is a God of healing and renewal. I stand firm in my beliefs that Jesus Christ is my Lord and Savior and my faith has been a dominating factor in how I feel physically and how I view things outwardly. I just have total reliance on God in my everyday encounter with this condition, thanking Him every day for every physical movement (i.e. walking, running, cooking, etc.) I am able to make that used to be a struggle in the past. So, this has made me more aware in appreciating all my abilities to move physically, think clearly and pray without ceasing.

Q: What role has nutrition, healthy living and exercise played in your life? Do you exercise or follow any specific eating habits? And, have you ever consulted with a nutritionist?

A: Nutrition, healthy living and exercise play an important role in the management of my condition because it helps promote a stronger sense of self and helps to boost bone strength and lower the risk of heart disease, which are both prevalent in lupus. The risk of developing osteoporosis and heart disease are high due to medication and the inflammatory process of the disease, respectively, so I find it important to maintain a healthy lifestyle. I enjoy participating in recreational activities such as swimming, bike riding and rollerblading. In regards to my eating habits, I include juicing raw vegetables and fruits. I try to consume a healthy portion of fish and big servings of fruits and vegetables daily, which helps to satiate my appetite and maintain my weight at a healthy number. I do notice eating certain foods such as chocolate does have a negative impact on my symptoms. Exercise has helped to elevate my mood and warm my muscles and joints, particularly Pilates and Yoga. I notice the importance of stretching is essential to stimulate blood flow to the muscle and bones, as well. Also, I take Ca++ tablets to increase bone strength again due to medication side effects, such as prednisone.

Q: How would you finish the following two sentences?
I am at my best and will continue to strive at my best in my faith...
Even with lupus, my life is all I have dreamed of...

A: I am at my best and will continue to strive at my best in my faith because I have come face to face with one of the hardest life challenges that has only made me stronger.

Even with lupus, my life is all I have dreamed of because I am at a point in my life where I am most content, peaceful and stronger than ever before.

Q: If your character, your life, your dreams, etc., could be summed up in one quote or motto, what would it be and why does it mean so much to you?

A: "Do you want to know who you are? Don't ask. Act! Action will delineate and define you," by Thomas Jefferson. After reading this particular quote by Thomas Jefferson, it resonates very profoundly in me that as long I am moving and acting towards my pursuits, things will align and will become sharper like the tip of a diamond. So, I like to think I'm in "sharpening" school.

Q: Who are the most important people in your life and why?

A: My mother, father, sister, brother and niece because most importantly they are a part of me. My mother possesses a quality of relentless love through her actions of giving and nurturing in ways only a mother knows how to. She is a treasure. My father has been a very strong-willed person in my life, silently praying and striving to make sure I am always okay. My sister, who is my very best friend and one of my greatest supporters, sustains me and holds me up when I am weary. And, I do the same for her. She has been by my side without any hesitation. My brother is someone who responds immediately when needed and would provide the voice of reason at the right time for me.

Q: *What are your plans for the future, despite lupus, and how do you plan to achieve them?*

A: My plan for the future is to continue and excel in my efforts to be one of the outstanding voices and advancing the efforts in health disease prevention and promotion. I also want to continue my volunteerism in the community and properly educate people in healthcare on a wider scope. Being an advocate in those things are very important to me and I feel needed there through my profession in medicine and public health.

Q: *What are three tangible pieces of advice that you would offer to someone struggling with the disease?*

A: First, learn about your medical condition via reputable sources such as www.lupus.org, through teleconferences, lectures, symposiums and reading materials they provide. Second, build your support system and stick very close to them, particularly those with lupus as well. There will be times when you just need to talk to someone and they will not only sympathize but empathize as well. Third, take your medications as prescribed. In addition, commit to attending your scheduled doctor's appointments. Be in constant communication with your specialist especially if you have a question about your condition, how to take your medication, and bringing up any new symptoms/signs you are experiencing. It is important to catch these early and attend to them.

Q: Last, please finish the following sentence:
Even though I was diagnosed with lupus...

A: Even though I was diagnosed with lupus, I have continued to stay more faithful and prayerful, in constant communication with God and show a more compassionate heart towards others. I celebrate every present moment by enjoying the gifts that are continuing to unfold in my life with positive, energetic people.

CHAPTER 4

The Story of Wendy D. Phillips

Miami, Florida
35 Years of Age
Educational Technologist –Educator

Q: Wendy, how you were diagnosed with lupus? What was happening in your life during that period, what age were you, and what type of symptoms were you experiencing?

A: Prior to being diagnosed in 2006, my family and I would joke that when I would have "flares," it was the lupus I was not yet diagnosed with. In 2005, I was diagnosed with cancer and during recovery I was not healing as well or as "on target" as the doctors thought I should be. In a nutshell, I was having severe setbacks that were unexplained. Several tests later they realized why I was not healing or recovering properly; I had lupus. Ultimately, I had strange side effects from the radioactive therapy that I was receiving to help me recover from cancer. Because of my compromised immune system, the lupus wreaked havoc on my organs and system. Lupus, over the next several months of 2006, proceeded to attack several of my major organs. Now, I was not only attempting to recover from cancer, but struggled with the lupus as well. At that time, I decided to change my career as an Elementary Teacher (ultimately, there too many germs I was being exposed to each day).

Q: How would you describe your initial reaction to the diagnosis? Were you somewhat expecting it or did it come as a shock to you?

A: Prior to being diagnosed, I knew I was a carrier. Lupus runs rampant in my family. My mother's paternal side of the family is where the lupus comes from. We have several people in our family that are living with lupus and have also passed away (both males and females) from complications of the disease. My mother had me checked when I was younger to see if my ANA levels were elevated and hoped lupus would never be "activated" in my body – especially at a young age. We normally would laugh at the small aliments, however as the symptoms became more and more pronounced by the time I was 28, my mother became more worried. The thought was, the younger you are when diagnosed, the shorter your life span is and the tougher it is on your body. I was also in the process of adopting a baby at the time I was diagnosed.

All though on the outside I was strong and portrayed a "Hey, I am invincible attitude," inside, I was scared. The reality was...who wants to die? There is so much to do in life; my bucket list had barely begun to be written, let alone be marked off.

Q: How does your initial reaction to the diagnosis differ from your outlook on life today?

A: Today vs. six years ago, there is a complete turnaround. My invincible attitude on the outside is now a reflection from the inside. During August of 2011, I was walking around Disney World on my 35th birthday, with a cane as I normally do, or in my wheelchair due to fatigue. Lupus likes to attack my legs, along with the majority of the left side of my body (strange, I know). Anyway, I decided to take the invincible attitude I once had prior to lupus and reestablish it. With my doctor's advice, I began an exercise regimen with the goal to run a 5K. After successfully running my third 5K, I met Jeff Galloway, Olympian, and had a wonderful conversation with him. This conversation inspired me to seek out more goals.

I then started training for a half-marathon. When I ran my first half-marathon, I met Kathrine Switzer, who was the first women ever to run the Boston Marathon (unofficially). She also helped to get women's marathon running into the Olympics. I spoke with her about the struggles that I personally had regarding health and such. As she is now a motivational speaker, needless to say, (even though she has not had much personal impact with lupus), her words of inspiration helped me to realize that lupus is just a simple test of strength and courage. This past year I ran four half-marathons, six 5K's, and four "Adventure Runs," thus far.

My outlook is I run because I can; I run for those who cannot. The funny thing is since I began running my health has improved. I can go to Disney without my cane, and without my wheelchair. I have more energy now than I have ever had. The key to me being able to keep moving is I listen to my body; when I am tired, I stop or slow down. I try not to push it even when my running buddies tell me I can go just a bit more. I remind myself they do not have to wake up with this body in the morning.

Q: What are some tangible lessons that you would like to share with a newly diagnosed person or someone who is struggling with the disease?

A: My biggest lesson I had to learn was to say, "No," even to my own mother. This was hard because she also has lupus. Also, taking time for myself, such as going to get my nails done – alone. The little things I like to call "quiet times." It is like putting yourself in shutdown mode or in "time out," you have to do this, otherwise you are on overload and that is when we are most likely to flare.

Taking naps, not really sleeping but just lying down on the couch and watching a movie or television, without doing anything else is helpful. Remember to do something for you. Again, it is about turning off your brain and relaxing.

Q: What has changed in your life because of the disease? Did you switch majors in college, perhaps quit your job and started a completely unrelated occupation, change your plans regarding having children, move to a different location, etc.?

A: I had to leave the classroom. At the time I was diagnosed, I was a classroom teacher. Between the excess amount of germs and the migraines, my doctors were worried that I would never be able to get my Lupus under control. I was put on FMLA leave for four months, after which I went back as a consultant for a vendor for the school board. I am still in the education field but not as a direct teacher. As for children, I realized that having children of my own would be extremely dangerous and selfish of me. Thus, I adopted. I want more children and would love to have my own; however, reason and logic remind me this would not be a likely scenario.

Q: What have you learned about yourself and your character through the lupus diagnosis? Has it made you stronger, more aware of taking care of yourself, or more compassionate?

A: I always knew I was a strong-willed person from the start. Lupus helped me learn how to compromise without compromising my goals and dreams. I finally figured out how to be a strong, independent woman, yet deal with the fact that I have a disease which sometimes makes me extremely dependent on others, and that does not compromise my integrity at all.

I always heard it takes a big person to ask for help. I never knew that more until I was confined to a wheelchair for over a year because of the lupus. Now, when I run, I appreciate each step. I even take the stairs every day. I realize that one day I was able to walk and the next day my own legs "betrayed" me and I could not function without the assistance of a wheelchair or other aids. The ability to be mobile is something I will never take for granted. I listen to a song with the lyrics, "What doesn't kill you makes you stronger," when I run. For most of my running buddies, I think they all think it is about the miles, however, I love that with each step I am moving. With each step, it is a reminder that I am winning my battle against lupus; with each step I am the victor thus far. And, with each step, it reminds me that not so far in the past lupus had me tight, but I am stronger now; we all are stronger.

Q: Do you consider yourself a fighter? What are some of the major hurdles you have had to deal with in terms of the disease? Think back to a moment you were very ill - how did you get to where you are now?

A: I have always thought of myself as a fighter even before I had lupus. However, I never really realized what the true definition of the word was until I was diagnosed with lupus. I thought a fighter was someone who was tough and never gave up. However, I realized that a fighter is someone who realizes his or her strengths and weakness, and realizes when it is time to ask for help. That is a true fighter,

My biggest hurdle was and still is asking for help. My second biggest hurdle is listening to my body and giving in. Sometimes it is almost like I am being defeated. But, then I remember the old saying, "You may have won this battle, but not the war." Then I laugh and I lie down and rest. It is my own personal joke. Some people do not get it. I love superheroes, so I sometimes think I am a twisted version of a superhero, like Super Girl...and my kryptonite is Lupus in a flare. It is the only thing that can keep me down. Yes, I am a geek, but it makes me laugh and I know tomorrow when I wake up I will feel better and will have a new day to kick butt!

As far as my sickest moments, there were two. When I was first diagnosed (2006) and about three years ago in 2009. In 2006, I began having horrible migraines that caused me to become bed ridden or hospitalized. It got to the point where my doctors decided that I needed to stop working; at that moment, we were waiting on my test results to come back. I was put on leave from work and eventually returned with a diagnosis of lupus. My doctors said I needed to be extra cautious and be sure to take all my preventative meds. Two years later, I was still suffering from horrific migraines and thus they put me on leave once more and told me I had to change careers. It was that or potentially have the lupus kill me. At that point, the lupus was not only attacking my brain constantly and causing migraines, but also started attacking my left lung and kidneys on a regular basis. I took my doctor's advice and changed careers. I became educational support and worked for an outside vendor.

The second major low in my lupus life came about a year and a half later, when I woke up for work one morning and I could not move. My legs literally were frozen. My left leg was in so much pain, I was crying. My tendons were inflamed to the point that they were tearing. Not realizing what was going on, I attempted to walk. In doing so, I actually tore part of my Achilles due to the over inflammation that was surrounding the tendon. I was rushed to the ER. Besides the Achilles, the doctors realized

I had several other issues happening. My lung was filling with fluid, my kidneys were not working properly, and my liver was "clogging up." Needless to say, that flare was severe - the worse I have ever had.

I was in the hospital for about a week and then home recovering for another six weeks. Luckily, I was able to work from home, but as my mom would later say, "You know she is sick when she does not even want to turn on her computer." I was then put in a wheelchair for the next nine months because my body had taken such a beating and I could not support my own self. I had to learn to rely on everyone around me. I had to learn to drive differently. And, I realized that people looked at handicapped individuals very differently. This was an extreme low point for me. When we went to Disney, I could not walk or run around with my daughter. I had to use a cane or use a motorized chair. I was married and had a Disney Fairy Tale wedding on The Disney Cruise Line Dream in May of 2011 and honeymoon at Disney – can you tell we are huge Disney fans? While there, I could not just walk around, I had to use my cane. In Aug 2011, we went to Disney for my birthday. I woke up on August 4th and we were going to have breakfast. My wife handed me my cane and I went to take it. I looked at her and said, "No, not any more. Things have to change. I cannot live like this anymore. I have run out of words, synonyms, for being tired. And, I am done. When we get home, I am going to start running, and I am done using the cane."

I ran my first 5 K at the end of August and crossed the finish line in a little less than an hour with a girl I met whose mother also has lupus.

Q: Wendy, tell me about your support system.

A: My support system consists of mother, who also has lupus, my wife (who is my best friend and the other mother of my daughter), my step-daughter, my daughter, and my grandmother.

Q: What would you tell a newly diagnosed person regarding the importance of having a support system?

A: Find people who will love you but who will be honest with you. You need honesty in your life. You do not need people who will be passive with you, especially if you are stubborn and hardheaded.

Q: Describe the positives in life even after a lupus diagnosis. What is your perspective on how you can lead a productive life even with the disease?

A: Every morning I wake up, I have conquered the lupus. Each day, when I stand up, I have beaten it. I used to think of all the things I cannot do anymore, but in reality, I can still do them, just in different ways. I can still be a mom – my daughter is adopted and she is the spitting image of me. I never ran before I had lupus, and now I have done four half-marathons this year alone. Life is not about the "I cant's" - it is about the "how can I get this done." I used to have a dance teacher when I was young who told me there was no such words as "I can't." I still believe that. I never thought of myself as an optimistic person, but I guess I am. Each day I breathe, it is a good thing. Every day I walk, life is good. Each day brings new and exciting adventures and I am not going to miss that, regardless of what lupus has in store for me. I will rest, but I will not miss this adventure I call my life because I have lupus, it is just too much fun.

Q: How does faith play a role in your disease? What are your beliefs and how have they helped you get through not only the difficult diagnosis, but also everyday hiccups that occur with lupus?

A: My belief in G-d has stayed strong. I grew up with the understanding that everything happens for a reason, and that G-d provides us with opportunities to make us a better person. Ultimately, this is a huge "test" if you will, but there are always those moments where one can just give up. I think that is what is being determined · the strength of our character. Do we just give up and allow this disease to control us, or do we decide that lupus is just a hitch-hiker that has decided to join our life and is along for the ride? I personally decided it is a hitch-hiker, that needs to, for the most part, follow my rules. Yes, once in a while "it" gets to determine when I rest, etc. However, "it" will not slow me down or decide that I am unable to achieve my dreams or goals in life.

Q: What role has nutrition, healthy living and exercise played in your life? Do you exercise or follow any specific eating habits? And, have you ever consulted with a nutritionist?

A: The only thing health wise I changed in my lifestyle is I began exercising. I started slowly with a run/walk Galloway Method training. From that, I worked my way up to a 1 minute run / 1 minute walk routine. Then I started weight training and swimming. I am now at a 3 minute run / 1 min walk routine and can run a 12 minute mile. This is my exercise. I run about four times a week · three short runs and one long run. My short runs consist of two, three and five miles runs, and one 5-7 mile run. My long run is usually a 10 – 15 mile run, depending on the week. During the season, from November through February, I was running about 30 to 35 miles a week. Food wise, I had to change my diet. As I lost weight, we realized I had a sugar problem; apparently, I am hypoglycemic. With all my running, I had to increase my carb intake and change my diet to a high-carb diet, 50% carbs, 25 % protein and 25% everything else. (I loved it). I lost about 40 pounds in my first few months because of running and dieting. I noticed that eating too much meat, beef, and processed food has a very negative effect on me. I try to stay away from foods with too many dyes, as they seem to make me feel "fuzzy." I will typically run across foods here and there that will "drain" me, typically beans. It seems weird, but all sorts of beans seem to make me sleepy or just foggy. Raw vegetables, especially celery and cucumber are great energy boosters, and good for dehydration. I eat these often as I also have Sjogren's syndrome.

Q: How would you finish the following sentence?
Even with lupus ...

A: Even with lupus, I know what my limits can be, however, I refuse to settle. I can work within and around those limits and still be all that I was meant to be and accomplish my dreams. I have seen too many people give up their hopes and dreams of living their life to the fullest because of lupus. Lupus is not a death sentence, but a life companion we must learn to compromise with sometimes. Through this disease, I have learned to be more humble, proud of who I am, and have more faith that G-d will allow me to have the strength to live out my dreams and be the person I was meant to be.

Q: If your character, your life, your dreams, etc., could be summed up in one quote or motto, what would it be and why does it mean so much to you?

A: "There are no such words ... 'I can't'"

Q: Who are the most important people in your life and why?

A: My mother, because she is a lupus warrior and is fighting the battle right along beside me. When she is sick, I hope I give her courage to keep fighting. On the flip side, when I am sick she is always right there for me. My wife, Jo; she is a huge supporter. She is always worried that I am over doing it when I run and very concerned that I will relapse. When I start to flare, she is usually the first to call me on it and tell me that I need to rest. My daughter would be the most important person and probably the reason I decided to take control of my lupus. I realized that when I was in the wheelchair, it was hard for me to push her in the stroller and I could not run after her. When I started walking again, it was still hard to play with her; I would take her to the park and just sit and watch her.

This past February, we ran three races together. It feels so good to be able to play with her, as a mother should.

Q: What are your plans for the future, despite lupus, and how do you plan to achieve them?

A: I just finished my Master's Degree and I plan to pursue my PhD. This year I have on my race list two full marathons and three half-marathons, on top of a few other races. I plan on going to California and running at Disneyland and getting my Coast-to-Coast Medal. I want to keep running for as long as I can. Next year, I plan on running in the New York Marathon, with Achilles International, which is a group for Disabled Athletes. I hope to begin raising money and awareness for lupus while I train for the NYC Marathon. One day, I hope to be able to run in the Boston Marathon with Switzer - that will be cool. I have created a 40 by 40 challenge for myself. The 40 by 40 challenge is for me to earn 40 medals that challenged me in some way by the time I am 40. I got the idea from others who ran a set number of marathons or half's by a set age.

My dream is to one day be on the podium in my age group, that would be way cool. As for my personal life, I was married last year - we have two children from previous relationships, however I would like to have another child. I think I am at the point that I really am enjoying life. So, I may rethink this. My 40th medal will hopefully be my original marathon, the Athens Marathon, that will bring me full circle, and then I will start again and perhaps begin a new challenge.

Q: What are three tangible pieces of advice that you would offer to someone struggling with the disease?

A: If something is not working for you and you do not feel right about it, seek out a different solution. I went through six rheumatologists before I felt comfortable with a game plan. Second, always take time for yourself, even if it is an extra 10 minutes in the shower to just breathe and let the rest of the world go away. It is not going to harm you or those you love. Remember if you do not take care of yourself, how can you care for those you love? And third, find something you are passionate about and do it. Just because you have lupus does not mean you have to give up your dreams; where there is a will there is always a way, find a way, go forth and be all you can be.

Q: Last, please finish the following sentence:
Even though I was diagnosed with lupus...

A: Even though I was diagnosed with lupus, I still live each day to the fullest. I appreciate every moment I have. I always knew I was strong person, however, living each day with the courage to overcome the obstacles that I face has proven that I am a woman of strength that surpasses even my own expectations sometimes. One of my favorite motivational songs when I run, that has also turned into one of my life's motivational songs, is by Miley Cyrus. I leave you with these words ... remember, life is what you make it, so make it a great! "Always gonna be an uphill battle; Sometimes I'm gonna have to lose. Ain't about how fast I get there; Ain't about what's waiting on the other side, it's the climb!"

CHAPTER 5

The Story of Damian Velez

Davie, Florida
36 Years of Age
Financial Analyst

Q: Damian, how you were diagnosed with lupus? What was happening in your life during that period, what age were you, and what type of symptoms were you experiencing?

A: The year was 1993. I was in my senior year of high school. I had never been sick before and I was very active in sports and other extra-curricular activities. I began to feel joint pain and stiffness early in the year, around February or March. I thought it had to do with my activities. It never occurred to me it might be something other than overdoing it in sports and exercise. The symptoms were so mild, I did not really give it any attention. I went to the doctor and was originally diagnosed with Juvenile Arthritis. About two weeks after my 18th birthday, my symptoms began to get worse. I would sleep all day and I had no appetite. Just the smell of food would make me nauseous. When I took a shower, the water hitting my skin would hurt me. This would result in my vomiting after every shower. I could not keep any food down. Every time I tried to eat anything, I would immediately throw it up. I went from weighing 185 lbs. to about 140 lbs. in less than a month. I went back to the doctor, and this time I was re-diagnosed with SLE. The doctor prescribed me a very small dose of prednisone. This seemed to aggravate my condition, and I quickly got worse. I would sleep 20-22 hours a day and I could not keep any food or liquids down at that point. My mother finally convinced me to go to the hospital where they quickly admitted me. I was severely dehydrated and was told if I had I waited any longer, I may have begun to experience organ failure. I stayed in the hospital for nine days and was being administered 40 mg of prednisone. Thus began my life with lupus.

Q: How would you describe your initial reaction to the diagnosis? Were you somewhat expecting it or did it come as a shock to you?

A: I was actually quite indifferent to the diagnosis when I originally received it. I did not really know how to react. I had never heard of SLE or lupus. I did not know anyone who ever had it. No one in my family could think of anyone within the family that may have had it. As I thought about the diagnosis more and more, I began to get upset. I could not understand how I could have a "woman's" disease. I began to wonder how this was going to change my life. What was I going to do if I could not play sports anymore? Could I die from this? Would I be able to go back to school? These questions raced through my head with no visible answers. I remember being very bitter when I was alone, but I would put on a fake positive attitude when I was around my family and friends.

Q: How does your initial reaction to the diagnosis differ from your outlook on life today?

A: I do not know how to fully answer this question. I have my good days and I have my bad days. Honestly, I still feel a tad bitter at having lupus.

Q: What are some tangible lessons that you would like to share with a newly diagnosed person or someone who is struggling with the disease?

A: It is hard to say. Learning to ask for help is definitely a big one. There comes a point in the life of someone with lupus where they realize they really cannot do it all by themselves, no matter how much they tell themselves they can. Surrounding yourself with caring and loving people is definitely a good start. Understand that with this disease, one has to live day by day. Some days are going to be better than others are, and that is alright. Just because one day or one week might be rough, that does not automatically mean there is a flare up in your near future or this is the beginning of the end.

Q: What has changed in your life because of the disease? Did you switch majors in college, perhaps quit your job and started a completely unrelated occupation, change your plans regarding having children, move to a different location, etc.?

A: I was diagnosed at a young age, so living habits had not really been established yet. Having health insurance became a number one priority. I made sure to choose jobs that were indoors and not labor intensive. I also chose jobs where they would be willing to work with me and my doctor's appointments.

Q: What have you learned about yourself and your character through the lupus diagnosis? Has it made you stronger, more aware of taking care of yourself, or more compassionate?

A: Having this disease has definitely made me more compassionate and understanding of other people's vulnerabilities and issues they might be facing on a day-to-day basis. It also caused me to be less judgmental of others. People have things going on in their lives that may cause them to be moody or anti-social, because they do not know of any other way to act. These are people that need to be shown there is a better way to react to things and that one can live with various issues without being bitter or angry all of the time.

Q: Do you consider yourself a fighter? What are some of the major hurdles you have had to deal with in terms of the disease? Think back to a moment you were very ill - how did you get to where you are now?

A: I do not really consider myself a fighter. I guess when I was younger and had no children I did not really care what happened to me. I never really kept to any regimented schedule when it came to my medicine. I would go to the doctor because I was told I had to in order to continue getting my medicine. I would say this is the biggest hurdle I had to deal with in terms of the disease - admitting that my life would never be the same. My sickest moment occurred shortly after I was diagnosed. The amount of prednisone I was being prescribed was not enough so I had a bad flare up. I lost a great deal of weight and was severely dehydrated. I was admitted into the hospital and had to stay there for nine days. I do not know if I would say this experience made me stronger, but it definitely made me realize this was something that was not going away and could potentially kill me if not kept in check.

Q: Damian, tell me about your support system.

A: My family is my main support system. They try their hardest to be supportive and understanding, but they are very emotional people. Every time they have ever seen me sick or in the hospital, it crushes them. They always seem like they are at a loss as to what to do or what to say.

Q: What would you tell a newly diagnosed person regarding the importance of having a support system?

A: Try to be understanding with your support system, whether it is family, friends, or co-workers. Try to remember, they more than likely have never had to deal with this and may not know the right or wrong things to say and do. Be patient with your support group. If they are willing to offer their support, accept it without being critical. If they are doing something incorrectly, point it out to them, but reinforce how appreciative you are for all of their help and support.

Q: Describe the positives in life even after a lupus diagnosis. What is your perspective on how you can lead a productive life even with the disease?

A: Provided you take your medicine regularly and do what you can to avoid the sun or strenuous activity, you should not really limit yourself in any other way. Make goals just like anyone else. Tell yourself just because someone is healthy does not guarantee they will accomplish all of their goals in their lifetime. The same goes for someone living with lupus; you may not be able to accomplish all of the goals you set out for yourself, but that does not mean you should not set them anyway. I feel setting goals helps keep me focused on doing more and accomplishing what I set out to do. This does not give me too much time thinking about how my life could be different if I did not have lupus.

Q: What role has nutrition, healthy living and exercise played in your life? Do you exercise or follow any specific eating habits? And, have you ever consulted with a nutritionist?

A: I have exercised in the past and I have attempted to eat nutritiously, but I am undisciplined when it comes to my eating habits. As for exercising, in college I participated in a number of intramural sport activities. I also played roller hockey within a league and regularly played basketball. After college, I had less time to exercise so I joined a spin class/gym, and regularly played paddleball with a friend. I found spinning to be the best workout, because it allowed me to have a great cardio workout without putting my joints through too much punishment. I have never seen a nutritionist, although I have wanted to for quite some time, and I do not really follow any specific eating patterns, because I become bored with the same foods very quickly. I have noticed that when I am heavier, due to eating poorly, my joints ache a little more from the extra weight. I would not say exercise has helped me manage the disease any better, but it does make me feel better about myself and about the way I look. Although exercising too much or too hard can cause me to flare up, it is difficult to determine how much is too much, because as with anyone, you want to see results as quickly as possible and it is very easy to overdo it.

Q: How would you finish the following sentences?
Living with lupus has caused me to be...

A: Living with lupus has caused me to be more aware of my body and any subtle changes that occur, which may or may not be signs of something more to come. I have also become more responsible when it comes to my social activities as a result of living with lupus.

Q: Who are the most important people in your life and why?

A: My immediate family members are the most important people in my life. I always know I can count on my mother and siblings for anything I might need or for support concerning anything I might be going through. Of course, there is also my daughter. She is the reason I wake up every day and persevere over anything I might be going through as a result of this disease.

Q: *What are your plans for the future, despite lupus, and how do you plan to achieve them?*

A: I plan to eventually purchase a house and place my daughter in a better school than the one she is currently attending. I plan to achieve these goals by continuing to work hard at my job, and trying to stay as healthy as possible.

Q: *What are three tangible pieces of advice that you would offer to someone struggling with the disease?*

A: Anyone struggling with this disease should make sure they are keeping the lines of communication between all of their doctors open, and make sure the doctors are actually talking to one another when it comes to treatments and medications. When visiting the doctor, remember to mention anything and everything you might be feeling or going through no matter how miniscule you think it might be. Let them decide whether it should be something to be concerned about or not. Lastly, always approach each day with as much of a positive attitude as you can. This will not always make your day brighter, but it will definitely help in making it seem less gloomy.

Q: Last, please finish the following sentence:
Even though I was diagnosed with lupus...

A: Even though I was diagnosed with lupus, I refuse to live my life wondering what this disease might do to me in the future, and I live each day knowing I can overcome whatever this disease might throw at me that day.

CHAPTER 6

The Story of Kathleen Walker

Hayden, Idaho
55 Years of Age
Insurance Agency Manager/ Self-published Author

Q: Kathleen, how you were diagnosed with lupus? What was happening in your life during that period, what age were you, and what type of symptoms were you experiencing?

A: I was diagnosed two years ago after a tumultuous year and a half of suffering. I had multiple overlapping symptoms that did not make sense to any of my doctors. I'd had a year and a half of crushing chest pain, shortness of breath, and pain all over my body but none as excruciating as the chest pain. Turned out, I had chronic recurring pericarditis, which helped the rheumatologist make the diagnosis when lupus finally showed up in the blood work. I also have rheumatoid arthritis and fibromyalgia, so I am considered a "crossover" patient.

Prior to the day I went to the ER for the first time with chest pain, I had not presented any definitive symptoms. For many years, my doctors scratched their heads at some mild symptoms I had that they could not pinpoint, i.e., skin problems, problems with menstruation, bladder control, and IBS. It was not until after I was diagnosed that it was all attributed to autoimmune diseases, most of it due to lupus. The RA causes swollen and painful joints, but lupus gives me much more grief than RA. Fibromyalgia is also very problematic and we are working on controlling that now. I was working (playing) at a side business I had that consisted of helping independent musicians get ahead in the business. I was doing booking and promoting and enjoying it very much. Music is a big love of mine and I was having a great time working with talented people I admired. I had just returned two weeks prior to my first ER visit with the excruciating chest pain from Chicago, where I helped organize a reunion of two musicians who had not played together in ten years. It was a fabulous time with great people and fantastic music. I just did not know it would be my last trip of that kind, so I am glad I went and got to have a great musical experience with people I really love.

Q: How would you describe your initial reaction to the diagnosis? Were you somewhat expecting it or did it come as a shock to you?

A: Initially, I was relieved when the diagnosis came. Finally, there was a name to describe what I was suffering from for a year and a half and enduring the doubt and snickers of the medical community. I actually had healthcare personnel say, "You look fine," so therefore I must be fine. I had this fantasy that once there was an official diagnosis, the Dr. would say, "Here's how we are going to make you all better." Of course, that did not happen. I take a plethora of pills and shots to stop the progression of the disease, but nothing helps the fatigue. I do not handle it well most of the time; I get discouraged.

Q: How does your initial reaction to the diagnosis differ from your outlook on life today?

A: I have learned to just live with it day to day. Some days, I can do just about anything I did before I got so sick and gained some weight. Other days, it is all I can do to lift myself out of bed and function in some fashion. I know there is no cure, unlike before I was diagnosed, when I believed I would be cured once there was a name. I believed that someone would give it a name, and viola! I would be made better by modern medicine. It is amazing to me how little the medical community still does not know about lupus. It is still a mystery disease to many healthcare professionals. My outlook is one of maintain and be positive, but I no longer hope for a cure.

Q: What are some tangible lessons that you would like to share with a newly diagnosed person or someone who is struggling with the disease?

A: First, learn to say, "No!" I have always been all things to all people and my family still expects it of me, even after I have explained to them how sick I really am. Since the damage occurs on the inside, it is difficult for them to imagine I do not feel as good as I look.

Second, rest is so important! Even if you feel okay and want to try to tackle difficult tasks, your body is deteriorating on the inside when you push yourself. I have to order others around to get household chores done. At first, I felt a little guilty about it, but when my body was telling me I could not do any more, I do not feel so bad about it now. I want to live longer, so I try harder to take care of myself.

Third, I know the meds have some undesirable side effects, but please do not think that just because they have helped you feel better, that you should give them up. Not true! Keep taking all the meds. I once went off Plaquenil because I thought I did not need it anymore, boy was I wrong. I will not make that mistake again.

Probably the most difficult part, while you are remembering to take all the medications, get plenty of rest, and get help for daily tasks, is to try to enjoy a little bit of each day without stressing. That is one of my biggest challenges. Getting over the pain, the limitation in my body, the chronic fatigue...I still try to find something that I enjoy doing every day. For me, it is writing. It is a productive outlet and gives me great satisfaction. And, it does not require a lot of physical exertion. I have also found a way to work with the bands I love and still do some booking and promoting for them; the internet is an amazing tool. I do a lot of it by phone, too, so I can do things to help others with something I enjoy at the same time. It is a win-win!

Q: What has changed in your life because of the disease? Did you switch majors in college, perhaps quit your job and started a completely unrelated occupation, change your plans regarding having children, move to a different location, etc.?

A: I did make some changes. I accelerated getting my books in print and on e-readers. I feared the diseases would take me before I was able to finish what I started. I was a writer before I got diagnosed, so I had several projects in the works. Before I got sick, I figured I had plenty of time to work on them. I started the process of self-publishing a lot sooner than before I was diagnosed.

Q: What have you learned about yourself and your character through the lupus diagnosis? Has it made you stronger, more aware of taking care of yourself, or more compassionate?

A: It has taught me to treat everyone with the same kindness and consideration I would want to be treated with because appearances can be deceiving. I have met a lot of people like me, who look okay on the outside, but on the inside are sick and diseased and struggle every day just to exist. It has brought out a softer side of me that I always had, but did not always show in my hurried work day. I have slowed down and I see little pleasures in life much more vividly. The flowers peeking up out of the dirt now that it is spring are fabulous! Little things like that, which I might not have noticed so much before, are important.

Q: Do you consider yourself a fighter?

A: Yes, I am very much a fighter. I personally know people who I feel would not be able to withstand what I have gone through. They would have ended up in the psych ward! I have always been the strong one in the family. My husband...not able to attend funerals, take care of sick kids, could not even change a diaper when the kids were babies. He would gag and barf. I had to do it all, and I did it without whining or complaining. Yes, I do pat myself on the back for that; somebody had to be strong.

Q: What are some of the major hurdles you have had to deal with in terms of the disease? Think back to a moment you were very ill - how did you get to where you are now?

A: Well, I know I have said it several times, but the fatigue is so overwhelming. I can shower and dress and then I just have to sit and catch my breath. It seems like I should be able to move my body and get up and *do* something, but I cannot. My body will not move and I have no choice about it. It is stifling, and it took me a long time to deal with that. Sometimes, I still do not deal with it too well. When I have a flare up, just holding a book up to read is too difficult, so sitting and watching TV or not doing much of anything is hard.

In the beginning, I honestly had days when I prayed for God to just take me home. I had chest pain so bad that pain meds did not touch it, and I ended up in the ER getting pumped up with morphine, which I hate. I felt so weak in my body and I was tired of fighting. I did not have the will to try to get better. Since I got diagnosed and on meds, I usually maintain somewhat of an equilibrium to my days, but I have had some awful flare-ups that make me realize (again) how sick I am and that I have to be extra vigilant. I try to take advantage of the good days and do what I can without overdoing it, but it is a fine line I cross sometimes when I get on a roll.

Q: Kathleen, tell me about your support system.

A: Well...that is a difficult subject. Because I have always been the strong one to hold everything and everybody together, it is difficult for my family to realize how sick I am. My children are all adults, but they are all healthy, so they have never experienced being very weak and sick. They bring me their stresses in their lives and early on, I would still try to help them "fix" whatever was wrong, but it took such an emotional toll on me that turned into a physical toll. Eventually, I had to take an "everybody has to take care of themselves" attitude. It is hard, even now.

My husband is in complete denial. Although the ER visits have become less, now that I have a treatment plan, I still have to try to tell him how sick I am. He sees me take pills every day and give myself the shots, he knows about all of my Dr. and lab appointments, but he will not believe I am truly sick until I end up in a hospital bed again. Then, he will be great about taking care of things for a few days until I am back on my feet. Then he will act as if everything is okay again. It is frustrating and it is not that I want sympathy; in fact, I go out of my way to discourage that.

Maybe that is a reason people do not realize how sick I really feel. I do not whine, moan, and complain about how bad I feel; I just go to bed and rest.

Q: What would you tell a newly diagnosed person regarding the importance of having a support system?

A: To be open, honest and do not spare *their* feelings! They are not the ones who are sick and need the support, so let them deal with their own reactions, on their own. You do not need to take that on yourself. Easy to say, right? I need to take my own advice.

Q: Describe the positives in life even after a lupus diagnosis. What is your perspective on how you can lead a productive life even with the disease?

A: Sheer determination is what it takes! It would be *so* easy to give up, stop doing anything and just sit around waiting for the end, but frankly...I would not be able to settle for that. I've always been an overachiever and I have always been a winner and I'll be darned if I am going to allow the illnesses to dictate to me!

Q: How does faith play a role in your disease? What are your beliefs and how have they helped you get through not only the difficult diagnosis, but also everyday hiccups that occur with lupus?

A: Faith is a subject I cannot really speak about. I come from a very dedicated fundamentalist Christian background, but honestly...my illness and pain has caused me to question a lot of that in recent times. I am still working on it, so I do not feel like I can advise anyone else.

Q: What role has nutrition, healthy living and exercise played in your life? Do you exercise or follow any specific eating habits? And, have you ever consulted with a nutritionist?

A: Exercise definitely helps. I walk very little, due to the RA, but even a little walk outdoors helps boost my mood and get the endorphins going. Anytime we can get up and move around, I believe we feel better. I can do water aerobics and that is very beneficial. Food most certainly is a big deal. I can tell when I do not follow good nutrition, my body feels like a big blob...just heavy and bloated, and it does not help my joints or my chest pain from the lupus. I do try to eat a balanced diet of all the food groups. I believe in everything in moderation and try not to go overboard on my favorite things, like brownies. Yum!

Q: How would you finish the following sentence?
In spite of all the pain and limitation...

A: In spite of all the pain and limitation, I think I have grown into a better person because I am more understanding and patient. I persevere even with limited physical strength because I do not want to let the disease take over; I want control over it.

Q: If your character, your life, your dreams, etc., could be summed up in one quote or motto, what would it be and why does it mean so much to you?

A: Never give up! Because if I had, I would not be of any benefit to others who need guidance and could benefit from my experiences.

Q: *Who are the most important people in your life and why?*

A: My rheumatologist, my youngest daughter (who I am closer to than just about anyone), and my mother, because she aches for me. She wishes she could take it all away and make me better, just as any mother would. She is one of the sweetest, most faithful women I know. She never wavers in her faith that God will heal all of this in His time, not ours.

Q: *What are your plans for the future, despite lupus, and how do you plan to achieve them?*

A: With meds to control progression, I plan to do just what I am doing now with the exception of working a day job. I have stayed at my day job to get through some financial hurdles due to my illness, and to help out my employer who has been amazingly good to me through it all. I want to retire by the end of the year. I qualify for disability; I just need to go through the hurdles of being able to get it. Then once I do not have to work a day job, I want to write full-time and get my next two books published. It is my joy! I would be able to spend more time with my family too, and that is a big motivation to stop working.

Q: *What are three tangible pieces of advice that you would offer to someone struggling with the disease?*

A: First, take care of *you* - that is most important. Second, take your medication! It is hard to get used to and some days, I am not sure I can swallow another pill or load another syringe, but the alternative is not a very attractive thought. Third, be honest with the people who care about you. You do not need to whine, or beg for pity, but honestly tell people how you feel and that you may not always look as bad as you feel, but still need a lot of rest and less stress. Keep life simple.

Q: *Last, please finish the following sentence:*
Even though I was diagnosed with lupus...

A: Even though I was diagnosed with lupus...I have not given up my dream of being a published author. It has been a struggle at times to keep up with all the work involved in self-publishing, but I have done it even with lupus. I think that it pretty awesome.

CHAPTER 7

The Story of Laurie Renfro

Atlanta, Georgia
47 Years of Age
Writer & Master's student of Transpersonal Psychology

Q: Laurie, how you were diagnosed with lupus? What was happening in your life during that period, what age were you, and what type of symptoms were you experiencing?

A: I was diagnosed at age nine after about a year of frequent stomach aches, low-grade fevers and the emergence of the Discoid Lupus "butterfly" rash on my face. I was in the fourth grade, living in a two-parent adopted family (one sister, also adopted) with everything on the surface appearing optimal. I was not adopted until I was four years old however, and from the age of six months until my adoption, I lived in several different foster homes. My Systemic Lupus diagnosis was not confirmed until I developed internal bleeding that put me into a coma.

Q: How would you describe your initial reaction to the diagnosis? Were you somewhat expecting it or did it come as a shock to you?

A: My diagnosis turned my life upside down. My simple, safe life as a little girl was effectively over. I do not recall being terribly afraid though. I believe being surrounded by a reassuring family, community and medical staff was key.

Q: How does your initial reaction to the diagnosis differ from your outlook on life today?

A: My outlook today is extremely positive despite my "on-paper" reality. Fortunately for me, "change" did not translate into despair.

Q: What are some tangible lessons that you would like to share with a newly diagnosed person or someone who is struggling with the disease?

A: Take care of the basics · eat well, rest well and exercise well. Your body will "tell" you if a prescription is not working for you, an activity is too much, too little or just right, an issue is worrisome, a relationship is nourishing, and just about everything else that matters in your life. Take advantage of instructional reading and bodywork practices, such as Yoga and Qi Gong, for an improved felt-sense of your body.

Also, do not neglect your mental health. There is strong evidence for psychological factors manifesting as physical symptoms and diagnoses. Take on a personal spiritual practice, let go of any fears about dealing with mental health professionals, and begin to see yourself as an advocate for your mental health.

Choose the people in your inner circle. If you are old enough to choose the people in your life, evaluate each for whether they bring stress, drama or negativity into your life. As well, look beyond your current circle for positive people you might add.

Also, stay away from vice and excess. Lupus puts more than enough challenges into your life. There is no room for smoking, drinking and drugs (including marijuana and prescription drugs not prescribed by your doctor).

Do not ignore symptoms. Symptoms should be "welcomed" for the information they provide. Dismissing or avoiding symptoms will leave you in the dark and a "sitting duck" for an eventual medical disaster.

Live in the present. Your life is happening right now - not in the past or in the future. It is easy to get obsessed with things you had planned to do and ways your life has changed, possibilities of drug related side effects, diagnosis potentialities and more. Doing this, however, only steals your opportunities to live in the moment.

Do not own the disease. I do not use possessive pronouns associated with Lupus. Saying "my disease" or "my Lupus" is a way of taking ownership. From your own mouth to your own ears, this verbal practice of ownership has a strong psychological effect and overall health and well-being.

Q: What has changed in your life because of the disease? Did you switch majors in college, perhaps quit your job and started a completely unrelated occupation, change your plans regarding having children, move to a different location, etc.?

A: While I am not sure it was entirely due to the lupus diagnosis, I am a very determined, positive and visionary person. I believe my intention can lead to reality. I am not afraid to lose and take calculated risks. The only thing I am certain has changed is I am no longer afraid of dying. Instead, the only thing I can call a fear is my feeling about missed opportunities for living. I recognize life is short whether you have lupus or not. We all do best when we treasure and take advantage of every opportunity to truly live.

Q: What have you learned about yourself and your character through the lupus diagnosis? Has it made you stronger, more aware of taking care of yourself, or more compassionate?

A: Lupus has taught me everyone must take responsibility for his or her own life. There are no special passes for people with medical issues, nor passes for people who are completely healthy. Quality of life is not a matter of what a person has or does not have, but is directly connected to a person's attitude and willingness to seek enrichment.

Q: Do you consider yourself a fighter? What are some of the major hurdles you have had to deal with in terms of the disease? Think back to a moment you were very ill - how did you get to where you are now?

A: I do consider myself a fighter and have made it through many challenges. "Making it," though, for me, does not necessarily mean returning to full health and functioning. Instead, "making it," means coming through the challenge with a clear understanding there is more for me to do in life. Some of the major hurdles I have had to deal with include recovery from seizures, internal bleeds and major and vascular surgery. I was diagnosed with kidney failure when I was twenty-nine, had a transplant and nephrectomy a few years later, and have been on several different dialysis modalities since. My optic nerve was damaged via oxygen deprivation in 2006 and I had to do a complete rehab in order to deal with initial blindness, then, significant visual impairment. I think my sickest moment was associated with Peritoneal dialysis, when my peritoneum became infected with a highly resistant bug.

Q: Laurie, tell me about your support system?

A: As a girl and young adult, my support system included my family, teachers, church community and medical professionals. As I became an adult, my support community expanded to include friends, my therapist and people associated with life affirming activities, such as meditation and yoga.

Q: What would you tell a newly diagnosed person regarding the importance of having a support system?

A: I would tell a newly diagnosed person they must have a healthy support system!

Q: Describe the positives in life even after a lupus diagnosis. What is your perspective on how you can lead a productive life even with the disease?

A: No one person's life is perfect. Even people who seem to have it all also have challenges that have the potential to destroy life. Once you stop complaining and comparing, life becomes ripe with opportunities for wondrous living. Your life is a gift and lupus can either be suffered through or it can be engaged for new possibilities. Of course, you most will likely need time and assistance to come to this conclusion. Opening yourself to professional resources beyond your doctor is vital to moving beyond where you are to where you would like to go.

Q: How does faith play a role in your disease? What are your beliefs and how have they helped you get through not only the difficult diagnosis, but also everyday hiccups that occur with lupus?

A: I grew up in a Christian household and did an average job of living according to Christian tenants until I was about thirty years old. At that point, my long-standing interest in spirituality took over. I have since studied many great faiths and include a variety of spiritual practices in my everyday life. I do not think it is important to believe in god or embrace any certain religion or practice. I do think, however, it is vital to connect to the Spirit of Life through personal seeking and practice for the fruits of discipline, availability and awareness.

Q: What role has nutrition, healthy living and exercise played in your life? Do you exercise or follow any specific eating habits? And, have you ever consulted with a nutritionist?

A: I have not always been good to myself. It has taken time, and unfortunately, consequences in order to learn some lessons. I now exercise at least twice a week, practice Yoga and follow a diet low in potassium and phosphorus (related to kidney failure). I have never felt the need to see a nutritionist but am well educated on the "do's and don'ts" of a good diet. I have not found any specific foods affecting symptoms. I eat what I like and keep an open mind to new foods.

Q: How would you finish the following sentence?
Even with lupus, ...

A: Even with lupus as a constant companion of sorts, my life has been incredible and promises so much more.
Lupus is not me and I am not lupus.

Q: If your character, your life, your dreams, etc., could be summed up in one quote or motto, what would it be and why does it mean so much to you?

A: "I am looking forward to a time everything brings me joy." – Maya Angelou. This quote speaks to me because of the intention toward joy. Intention is so very powerful and while Ms. Angelo may never find everything bringing her joy, her intention will direct her availability for joy and her own expenditure of energy and spirit toward that end.

Q: Who are the most important people in your life and why?

A: My two daughters (ages 26 and 21) and my girlfriends are the most important people in my life. Each of them, in their own uniquely special ways, fully chooses me. This intentional choice is the force empowering their availability, compassion and honesty. Their presence in my life calls me to my best.

Q: What are your plans for the future, despite lupus, and how do you plan to achieve them?

A: I am currently writing a novel and completing the first of a two-year Master's program. I plan to publish, speak and, perhaps, teach some aspect of Transpersonal Psychology. I am also fulfilling a wish to find joy in travel. My first solo travel adventure since I lost a significant portion of my eyesight back in 2007 is scheduled for October of this year. I will attend the four-day Dodge Poetry festival in Newark, New Jersey.

Q: What are three tangible pieces of advice that you would offer to someone struggling with the disease?

A: First, you can do more than survive; you can thrive. Second, be more afraid of not living than you are of dying. And third, do not quit your day job.

Q: Last, please finish the following sentence:
Even though I was diagnosed with lupus...

A: Even though I was diagnosed with lupus, I am a happy person and my life is amazing.

CHAPTER 8

Perspective Highlight: A Mother's Point of View

By Pat Huron, the Author's mother

I will never forget the day that my daughter was diagnosed with lupus. I was stunned and numb. I really knew nothing about the disease although I had heard of it. At least now we had an answer to what was causing all the symptoms and sickness. But knowing did not bring relief, just more concern about what lupus actually is and how my daughter was going to be affected by it.

We were not prepared for the journey we were about to take, but the good news is that we have survived some nasty episodes. We also learned a lot about the disease, the prescribed medications, on-going research, the attitudes and perspectives of our doctors and our own ability to be our best advocate and look for answers for our self.

Be assured and aware that lupus will test your endurance, provoke your patience, mock your intelligence and vex your spirit. Another sad reality is that doctors do not have all the answers, and research on the disease is in its infancy. Lupus is not a well-known disease among the populace and it needs a "face" to attract attention and bring in donations for research. Lupus, like any other disease, is a challenge to body, mind and spirit, but with the right attitude and answers, lupus can be overcome. The question remains: "Are we up to the challenge?"

One of the things we heavily researched and sought professional council for was nutrition and natural medicine. Our goal was to create a strong, healthy and sustainable physical body for my daughter. This would give her an edge in fighting the ravages of disease. Another important goal was exercise to strengthen the body, but this was harder to achieve when my daughter was too sick or weak to engage in much physical activity. We always strive for balance and listen to the body when it is calling for rest.

Coping with the emotional ravages of lupus is also demanding. My daughter was in nursing school at the top of her class when she fell ill. She was devastated when she learned that she could not continue her studies and had to relinquish her dream to practice medicine. Her body just collapsed under the weight of the disease and she did not have the strength or stamina to continue on her chosen path. She cried plenty but she finally realized that she had to accept reality and let go of her dream. We had quite a few "pity parties" as my daughter let go of many activities her friends were involved in (that she could no longer partake of) – like kick-boxing, dancing, gym workouts and holding down a full-time job. She also pondered about future dreams of marriage and having children. We are people of faith and it was our faith that helped us keep things in perspective and trust God to see us through every valley. Looking back now, it seems so long ago because my daughter has come a long way. She is regaining her strength and stamina. She has been blessed with a wonderful writing career. She has taken charge of eating healthy, keeping as active as possible, and socializing. She has also married a wonderful man and they have hopes of having a child sometime in the future.

The best advice I can give to any mother who has a child with lupus is to be there for them physically, emotionally and spiritually. There will be good days and bad days. You know your child better than most and you will know what they need at any given moment. You are their best advocate and may advise them regarding medical options – when to say "Yes" and when to say "No." You are also their coach and cheerleader. Encourage them to get back on track if the need arises. I would also recommend that you do your own research. There is so much available online regarding medical reports and journals. I found a lot of information on adverse effects of medication from European sources because of socialized medicine, which created a history of documented information. I also combine seemingly unrelated things with lupus in my searches to see if there are connections. It is amazing what you will find if you only look for it. Certainly last but not least, don't ever give up! Stay strong and stay focused, especially when your child cannot.

CHAPTER 9

The Story of Linda Bernal Apgar

Fort Lauderdale, Florida
Late 50s
Independent Contractor (Accounting and reception
assignments)

Q: Linda, how you were diagnosed with lupus? What was happening in your life during that period, what age were you, and what type of symptoms were you experiencing?

A: I was diagnosed about 15 years ago. The symptom was an elbow pain that would not go away. As is often the story with lupus, I went from doctor to doctor, getting different diagnoses and treatments. After a while, I am sure I was looked at as a hypochondriac and after a while, I was convinced I was. Eventually, I went to a rheumatologist who questioned if I had lupus since none of the treatments were working. He ordered blood work, which showed there were borderline markers for possible lupus - but nothing definite. But, once again I was sent on my way without an answer. Finally, I found a rheumatologist who specialized in autoimmune diseases and who took my symptoms seriously. He immediately saw the butterfly rash and recommended that I get a skin biopsy. Even then, the dermatologist who did the biopsy said it was a waste of time, since she did not believe the rash looked like the characteristic "butterfly rash." (Again, I started to wonder if I was crazy!) But indeed, the skin biopsy confirmed I had lupus – the mystery was solved and confirmed that "it wasn't all in my head."

If I had not found the rheumatologist who specialized in autoimmune diseases (many rheumatologists concentrate on arthritis), I feel I still would be misdiagnosed.

It took me a total time of two years to be diagnosed, and only because I was persistent, did not give up and drove every doctor crazy, questioning their diagnosis when nothing was getting better.

Q: How would you describe your initial reaction to the diagnosis? Were you somewhat expecting it or did it come as a shock to you?

A: I really did not know that much about the disease. The only reference I had was the fact that 15 years prior, a coworker had lost her sister to lupus. She had been in and out of the hospital and had died from kidney failure. I sunk into a major depression, not knowing how my life was going to change and what would be my future. I felt completely alone and isolated, believing that no one understood what I was going through. As with so many people who have lupus, I look healthy, which isolates you even more .It is hard for people to understand when you do not look sick. It took about six months before I started to feel there was a future for me.

Q: How does your initial reaction to the diagnosis differ from your outlook on life today?

A: I attacked the disease by becoming proactive - reading about the disease, becoming informed, finding out that it is not necessarily a death sentence (after I cried for two weeks). Now I know my limitations. I live in Florida and stay out of the sun as much as possible (which is hard, considering I live in the "sunshine state"). I know that stress is a major factor in causing flares. I had a very bad flare during an incredibly stressful time in my life. As a result, I try to avoid stress as much as possible and honor my health. My husband and I have also become very involved with the Southeastern Florida lupus chapter.

Q: What are some tangible lessons that you would like to share with a newly diagnosed person or someone who is struggling with the disease?

A: Become informed about the disease. Become proactive. Read up about lupus. There are support groups when you are ready. Be kind and patient with yourself when you are first diagnosed. Realize that all the emotional steps you go through (denial, depression, anger) are completely normal. Do not hide from the disease or feel ashamed. I am incredibly open about the fact that I have lupus. Many people do not even know what lupus is. I educate them. In turn, very often I find that so many people know people who do have lupus. It is amazing!

Also, eat well. Nutrition is so important. In addition, learn how to relax · meditation, Yoga, Pilates, etc. Be kind to your body. It is your temple.

Q: What has changed in your life because of the disease? Did you switch majors in college, perhaps quit your job and started a completely unrelated occupation, change your plans regarding having children, move to a different location, etc.?

A: I avoid the sun during peak hours. Fortunately, I have a job (independent contractor) that allows me to set my own schedule. I am much more aware of symptoms and I take them seriously when they occur. I also see my lupus physician and have lupus blood work done on a trimonthly basis.

Q: What have you learned about yourself and your character through the lupus diagnosis? Has it made you stronger, more aware of taking care of yourself, or more compassionate?

A: I have always considered myself a strong person but having lupus has made me appreciate each day and my health. Now I take good care of myself and try to remain as stress free as possible. In our home, I have little "mediation" areas. I also listen to my body and am religious in regards to medical care.

Q: Do you consider yourself a fighter? What are some of the major hurdles you have had to deal with in terms of the disease? Think back to a moment you were very ill - how did you get to where you are now?

A: Yes, I am a fighter. One of the major emotional hurdles was acceptance. I found that reaching out to others who are going through the battles of lupus was extremely helpful and I knew I was not alone. I have been fortunate that the disease has not attacked my internal organs but has affected mainly my skin, scalp and mouth (ongoing mouth sores).

Q: Linda, tell me about your support system.

A: Most importantly, I have my husband who is extremely supportive and compassionate. I have my bad emotional hours (and days) and he accepts me through all the highs and lows. I have good doctors (especially my lupus doctor) who understand the limitations of lupus. I also have a tremendous network of friends. However, no one understands the disease like those who have it; now I have some friends (who are going through the same struggles) to lean on.

Q: What would you tell a newly diagnosed person regarding the importance of having a support system?

A: Support system is a priority. The first support system has to be yourself. However, you must have people you can count on when you are going through a rough period. In addition, I think it is important to reach out to others who have lupus. Only they understand what it is truly like to have this disease.

Q: Describe the positives in life even after a lupus diagnosis. What is your perspective on how you can lead a productive life even with the disease?

A: When one is faced with difficult times in life, one has two choices. The first is to let the situation overwhelm you and control your life. The second choice is to confront the "situation" (i.e.: lupus), eventually accept it (this will take time), and appreciate life.

Q: How does faith play a role in your disease? What are your beliefs and how have they helped you get through not only the difficult diagnosis, but also everyday hiccups that occur with lupus?

A: I have always had a strong spiritual belief, which has helped me get through extremely difficult periods in life even before I was diagnosed. I believe that I have an angel who holds me when I feel those moments of despair.

Q: What role has nutrition, healthy living and exercise played in your life? Do you exercise or follow any specific eating habits? And, have you ever consulted with a nutritionist?

A: I have always believed that good nutrition is fundamental in maintaining a healthy life for everyone. I have always followed a good nutritional plan - even before I was diagnosed. I rarely eat sweets and base my "diet" on a lot of fruits and vegetables. I buy fresh fruit (that is in season) and then freeze it. Every day I prepare a smoothie using frozen fruit, juice and Greek yogurt. I also add flax seed, goji, and sunflower seeds. I take a multivitamin and other supplements (including Iron and Calcium) every day.

Exercise has been a part of my life since my early twenties. I still exercise even if I have to force myself out of the house. I have an iPod and if I cannot get myself motivated, I listen to some dance music before exercise and all of a sudden, I feel the motivation to work out. I love to dance and take Zumba classes. I feel that exercise is not only good for your body but also for your mind. If I have a stressful day and then work out, the stress just melts away. I have been fortunate enough that I can still exercise.

Meditation and relaxation technique are two other elements that are fundamental in learning to cope with lupus.

Q: How would you finish the following sentence?
Lupus has given me...

A: Lupus has given me a gift · I appreciate every day I have and who I have become. I do not let lupus determine who I am.

Q: If your character, your life, your dreams, etc., could be summed up in one quote or motto, what would it be and why does it mean so much to you?

A: I have always loved the saying, "I complained I had no shoes until I met a man who had no feet." It has been a motto that has been my rock through my life. No matter how tough things become, there is always someone going through a more difficult time and it puts things in perspective. The most beautiful reward is helping others and reaching out to those less fortunate. I was a social worker for twenty years and I am proud of the fact that I gave so much back.

Q: Who are the most important people in your life and why?

A: First, it would be my husband for his support, love and having the ability to make me laugh after all these years. Unfortunately, I do not have family locally. I have a close relationship with my brother in Colombia - he is a physician. So, I can count on him for "telephone consults." My friends are my rock. This is especially true with my long-term friends, who know and understand me so well.

Q: What are your plans for the future, despite lupus, and how do you plan to achieve them?

A: My dream would be to relocate to an area that is not as hot and sunny as southern Florida - especially in the summer. Of course, my ultimate dream would be to move to Northern California. I feel the lifestyle in that area is one that I can feel a part of.

Q: What are three tangible pieces of advice that you would offer to someone struggling with the disease?

A: This might be somewhat repetitive but to summarize where my journey has led me to, I believe you must educate yourself on lupus. Knowledge is power - not only for yourself, but for when you need medical advice. Lupus is a very complicated disease that can affect almost every organ of the body. The more knowledge and in touch you are with your body, the more aware you will be when you are developing a flare.

Also, learn to handle stress - through meditation, walks surrounded by nature, relaxation techniques, etc. Take an hour a day to unwind - just for yourself. Lean on others for support; you are not alone. When you are ready, reach out to others who have Lupus; they can be your lifeline.

Q: Last, please finish the following sentence:
Even though I was diagnosed with lupus...

A: Even though I was diagnosed with lupus, I still have a full and beautiful life. I am truly blessed!

CHAPTER 10

The Story of Nicole H. Francis

Port Saint Lucie
37 Years of Age

Q: Nicole, how you were diagnosed with lupus? What was happening in your life during that period, what age were you, and what type of symptoms were you experiencing?

A: I was 21 years old, well into my third year as an undergraduate student and I had two episodes of Iritis when an eye specialist told me I should see a rheumatologist. The doctor believed I could be dealing with a possible autoimmune disorder. I did not understand what he was saying and did not understand what an autoimmune disease was at the time. I had to have steroids injected into both eyes, because that second Iritis flare-up was so bad. He explained to me, as best he could, what an autoimmune disease was and how it affects the body.

After two weeks, my eyes were back to normal; months went by and everything seemed fine. Then, one day while leaving school to catch the sub-train (I was living in Chicago during that time), the last thing I remember was reaching into my pocket for my transit tokens and looking down to count the loose change in my hand that was mixed in with the transit tokens. The next thing I knew, I was at the bottom of those subway stairs. I must have passed out for a bit. Luckily, there was a nice woman who held my hand until the paramedics arrived. I was so glad she stayed with me, because I was crying and scared. Long story short, that was my first flare, and about three weeks after that incident, I was diagnosed with Systemic Lupus.

Looking back now, I had all the major symptoms. I just brushed them off as me over working my body – I was trying to graduate on time, be a good mother to my daughter Alicia, then just 3 years old, trying to take care of a household, and working part-time, while my husband worked full-time. I had major hair loss, joint pain and swelling, headaches that would last for days, and exhaustion, no matter what I did. I somehow managed to graduate, obtaining my BA that following year, after my diagnosis.

Q: How would you describe your initial reaction to the diagnosis? Were you somewhat expecting it or did it come as a shock to you?

A: At the time, I was so young; it did not soak in until ten years later. Seriously, I pretended for ten years that everything was okay, because those close to me were also having trouble dealing with my diagnosis. I did not attend my first support group until nearly eight years after my diagnosis, so the shock did not come until years later. I am at times still feeling the effects of that shock.

Q: How does your initial reaction to the diagnosis differ from your outlook on life today?

A: When I am "okay," I feel as though I can take on the world. I try to accomplish as much as I can for my family and keep my spirits up. I value life to the highest degree, and was this way even before I was diagnosed. It just makes me cherish it a bit more.

Q: What are some tangible lessons that you would like to share with a newly diagnosed person or someone who is struggling with the disease?

A: First, I will tell them that it is okay to acknowledge the pain, mentally and physically, and to not be too hard on yourself about what you were able to do before lupus turned your life "around and upside down." I would say, ask for help · even if it is not where you want it to come from, like family, (if they cannot or do not want to support you), reach out to the LFA, ALR or The SLE Foundation.

You cannot let frustration build up inside, as it will only make the illness worse. I would tell them to find an outlet· use a talent you were given to help you heal; use it to "scream"; use it to "communicate"; and use it to "cleanse" your spirit from all of the negatives. Learn to laugh and pamper yourself. Also, find out all about your disease and what your triggers are. Try to rest your body, eat more fruits and veggies, and for those of us on high doses of prednisone, try to avoid processed foods.

Q: What has changed in your life because of the disease? Did you switch majors in college, perhaps quit your job and started a completely unrelated occupation, change your plans regarding having children, move to a different location, etc.?

A: Yes, this was hard for me and I am still dealing with it · my job/career. I loved what I did and I worked with my company for nearly ten years before I had to stop. I moved to Florida, yes, for the better weather and for a promotion.

Q: What have you learned about yourself and your character through the lupus diagnosis? Has it made you stronger, more aware of taking care of yourself, or more compassionate?

A: Lupus has taught me that I am surly stronger that I give myself credit for. I did not realize how much I have gone through and pulled through, since my initial diagnosis. I was always compassionate · but lupus opened my eyes to who really cares and who does not.

Q: Do you consider yourself a fighter? What are some of the major hurdles you have had to deal with in terms of the disease? Think back to a moment you were very ill · how did you get to where you are now?

A: I believe anyone dealing with a debilitating illness, such as lupus, is a "fighter." You have to be· to help your body understand how important your own life is. There were so many sick moments · when I could not button up my shirt, put on my jeans, nor tie my own shoes...I will say that was a pretty low point. However, you have to push, push, push for the things you want, even if you have to find a different way to do to it.

Q: Nicole, tell me about your support system.

A: My writing is usually all I have, that seriously keeps my mental state stable enough to deal with the surprises that lupus brings. My daughter, husband and my son help to keep my spirits up, but for the most part, it is my writing that cradles me with support. It is truly amazing what our talents and gifts can bring out of us. And lastly, the LFA support group I attend.

Q: What would you tell a newly diagnosed person regarding the importance of having a support system?

A: I would tell them to go when they are ready. Do not allow anyone to tell them that they should or should not go, and do not allow someone to tell you that all support groups are negative.

Q: Describe the positives in life even after a lupus diagnosis. What is your perspective on how you can lead a productive life even with the disease?

A: Laugh, laugh and laugh! If I did not have such a massive sense of humor, I believe lupus would have "taken me under" mentally, a long time ago.

Q: How does faith play a role in your disease? What are your beliefs and how have they helped you get through not only the difficult diagnosis, but also everyday hiccups that occur with lupus?

A: Spirituality is an individual thing, as we all know. Find what gives you peace of mind, keeps you positive, or helps you snap back to reality quickly during and after a flare up. It takes great courage to wake up to lupus. We have to be spiritually, physically and mentally strong to "fight" through the dark days.

Q: What role has nutrition, healthy living and exercise played in your life? Do you exercise or follow any specific eating habits? And, have you ever consulted with a nutritionist?

A: I cannot work out as I use to but I think it plays an important role in our overall confidence. Also, eating right helps to keep down some of the disease symptoms and medication side effects.

Q: If your character, your life, your dreams, etc., could be summed up in one quote or motto, what would it be and why does it mean so much to you?

A: As a poet, I have written the following quotes that mean a lot to me: "Flying with broken, 'inexperienced wings', takes great determination (when you are first diagnosed). Even though the course end seems longer than you anticipated, life shall reward you with stronger 'wings' (with each flare, we get stronger), allowing you great access to 'higher views.'"

"When The Wolf is knocking, I just turn the music up louder." – I love music, and it helps along with my writing to get me through each day.

Q: Who are the most important people in your life and why?

A: My husband, daughter, son, parents, sister and brother · family means everything to me.

Q: What are your plans for the future, despite lupus, and how do you plan to achieve them?

A: I want to start running again, at least three days out of the week, and be more supportive of myself. I know, this may sound silly, but if I do not believe in myself, I might as well give up now. I want to write more, like I used too. I also want to travel and visit Italy and the United Kingdom.

Q: What are three tangible pieces of advice that you would offer to someone struggling with the disease?

A: Take care of yourself. Love each minute of each hour. Laugh and do not be so serious. Most importantly, know that you are beautiful, despite what lupus has done.

Q: Last, please finish the following sentence:
Even though I was diagnosed with lupus...

A: Even though I was diagnosed with lupus, I have become a stronger, more compassionate person and I will continue to fight this disease. I will live a wonderful life and continue to 'ride' my sense of humor, share my love and show others how to grow spiritually, even though their bodies are weak. My strong "spirit" can and will carry me far.

CHAPTER 11

The Story of PJ Nunn

Waxahachie, Texas
55 Years of Age
Publicist by trade, Psychologist/Criminologist by degree

Q: PJ, how you were diagnosed with lupus? What was happening in your life during that period, what age were you, and what type of symptoms were you experiencing?

A: In 2009, my family was in a financial crunch because my husband lost his job and we had to downsize to an old house. I did not realize it mattered, but several months after moving in, both my oldest son and I developed sinus infections that would not go away. A few months later after a bad storm, the ceiling caved in from a roof leak and we found the house was infested with black mold. Knowing there was no way the owners would be able to quickly remedy the situation I immediately began looking for a place to move, but was feeling so worn down by the infection I would find myself falling asleep at my desk in the middle of the day.

I found a house to lease and managed to move, despite the fact that my husband and I had separated by that time and I and my oldest son, then 30, were quite ill. My oldest daughter and youngest son and some friends helped us get our things moved and we settled in thinking now that we were away from the black mold, we would start feeling better. Unfortunately, that did not happen. I was hopeful for a few months, but my son just kept getting worse and ended up in the hospital in January 2010. By then, I was only able to work a few hours a day and my business was failing. My husband and I had reconciled and he had a job, but lost it in January due to business being slow (he was a car salesman). My son got increasingly worse. They identified a staph infection and severely weakened immune system that ultimately resulted in his kidneys failing, having his teeth pulled (the infection got into the jawbone), and finally his right leg amputated above the knee.

I was horrified at what was happening to my son, but was so sick myself that I could hardly leave my room. The entire year of 2010, I did not leave my house except to go to the doctor, to the ER or to the hospital twice to visit Dave, who was hospitalized seven of the 12 months. Each time I went to the Dr. or ER, I was told it was stress, bronchitis, or a sinus infection, and given an antibiotic. One morning I awakened around 4:30 a.m. with chest pains so severe I just knew it was a heart attack and called an ambulance. That was the first of several times they ran me through all the heart tests only to come to the same conclusion. My heart was fine; it must be stress.

Things continued to get worse. I could not get up if I fell on the floor. I could not stand long enough to shower and had to take a chair into the shower stall. Much of the time,

I could not even walk to the bathroom without help. There were bad days and worse days, but no good days. This continued through 2011 until summertime when I wanted to attend a birthday party being held at a park. Determined to go, my middle son helped me get there. I honestly did not think I would make it walking from the car to the picnic table, just a few yards away. I envisioned passing out and just laying there. Thankfully, that did not happen but I knew I had to get help somehow at this point.

Two weeks later, we got notice of eviction from our house. Without my income (I had stopped being able to work at all in June) and my husband's lack of income (all he had managed to get was a part-time job at a grocery store) we'd already had to surrender our truck and had no vehicle, and now we could not keep up with the rent. I knew there was no way I would have the strength to get anything packed or help find a place to live without getting some antibiotics, so I found a ride to the ER. The doctor there acted as if I was an annoyance coming there with a sinus infection until he saw the results of my labs, at which time he cursed out loud and a whole group of people suddenly surrounded me and made haste to have me admitted. I heard words like "leukemia" and "HIV." I was terrified, but too tired to care.

I ended up in the hospital for three weeks and had six blood transfusions during that time, as well as a large battery of tests. They ruled out many things, but nobody seemed to know what it was I had. Finally, I was able to wrestle a possible diagnosis out of the oncologist/hematologist who was seeing me. Maybe, just maybe, it was lupus. He could not diagnose it – for that I needed to see a rheumatologist. But, being a small town hospital, they did not have one. In fact, I found out later there was not one even near the town. When the social worker finally found one who was taking new patients and would see me on a payment plan, he was about an hour away and the earliest appointment he had available was almost three months away. Still, they had started me on prednisone, which made me feel so much better. That medicine stabilized my white blood count and hemoglobin count, so I felt hopeful.

Q: How would you describe your initial reaction to the diagnosis? Were you somewhat expecting it or did it come as a shock to you?

A: I was so relieved to finally have a name for what I was experiencing and to know that while it is incurable, it can be treated and managed fairly well. Especially, when the doctor said he believed the lupus symptoms were caused by my blood pressure medication, hydralazine, and that once that was out of my system, the symptoms would go away. So, I kind of had lupus, but not really, or so it seemed. That did not turn out to be the case, but it was a hopeful place to be for a while.

Q: How does your initial reaction to the diagnosis differ from your outlook on life today?

A: I am still more in the dark than I want to be, and not as optimistic as I once was. I have been living with these symptoms for more than three years now and while treatment makes me able to function a lot better than I did for a while, I still cannot do a lot of things I should be able to do at my age and it is discouraging. I have to fight harder for an optimistic outlook, often simply because so many medical personnel (like my PCP and the ER personnel) do not have a clue about lupus or what to do with it.

Q: What are some tangible lessons that you would like to share with a newly diagnosed person or someone who is struggling with the disease?

A: The very first thing I would suggest is to get hold of a local chapter of a lupus organization and connect with someone who has lupus and still maintains a positive attitude. I have made the rounds of the message boards and see two distinct types; those that encourage and inform, and those that commiserate and whine. You do not want the latter.

Secondly, make sure you are seeing a rheumatologist who regularly treats lupus and makes you feel comfortable. Treating lupus should be a team effort with both of you involved.

Q: What has changed in your life because of the disease? Did you switch majors in college, perhaps quit your job and started a completely unrelated occupation, change your plans regarding having children, move to a different location, etc.?

A: It honestly has not changed my life in that tangible a way, although it has definitely affected my "overdrive" mentality and made me set limits for myself. It has also made me more aware of the need for retirement planning, taking care of things that are important to me, knowing that physically I may not hold up as well as I would like. It has made me much more aware of my health and weight struggles. I have also started keeping what I call a "Life Book." It is just a scrapbook, but with some extras in it. I am making one for me, but I am also making smaller versions for each of my children. Sometimes I add photos and tags, other times I may just jot down a note, or save a shower invitation or a monogrammed napkin, or the wrapper of a favorite candy bar. Maybe it is the illness, maybe my father's recent passing, but I want to be sure they have tangible memories of our time together when I am not with them anymore.

Q: What have you learned about yourself and your character through the lupus diagnosis? Has it made you stronger, more aware of taking care of yourself, or more compassionate?

A: I think I have always been strong, but throughout all of this with myself and my son, I believe my priorities have shifted somewhat and I have learned to be a little more protective of my boundaries. My husband thinks my "Life Books" and my altered outlook are a little morbid and they definitely make him uncomfortable. Do not get me wrong · I am not in some kind of death mode and always thinking about it. Actually, I think I have become a little more accepting and realistic. I see the difficulties my mom has experienced with my dad's death, even though we had been expecting it for quite a while. I just want to be sure that if something happens and I die sooner than expected, I have left things in neat enough order to make it easier for my family. I am only 55 and have no plans to "check out" for many years to come, but I take pleasure in the feeling that I am planning for that eventuality by preserving memories my grandchildren might be curious about one day.

Q: Do you consider yourself a fighter? What are some of the major hurdles you have had to deal with in terms of the disease? Think back to a moment you were very ill - how did you get to where you are now?

A: I am absolutely a fighter. And, I am glad that my parents raised me with that quality. So many times it would have been easy to just accept what a doctor said as law and get completely discouraged, but when they would pronounce something as factual that was not good news, I automatically refused to just accept it without further investigation. Often it turned out not nearly as bad as first suspected. The more I have learned about lupus, the more I see the medical profession just does not know. That does not make them stupid, it just means there is still a lot that no one knows about regarding the workings of this disease and just because something happened a certain way once, does not mean it will always work that way.

Q: PJ, tell me about your support system.

A: I love my family – my kids, my husband, my mom and my siblings. None of them have a good understanding of lupus. Most of the time, my mom and siblings, because I do not see them often, do not even think I am ill. My husband and my sons that live at home know I am not well, but even they do not really think of me as sick. They just think my knee hurts and I have to use a cane, or some days I do not feel good. My PCP is a very caring woman and wants to help, but she is visibly relieved when I tell her the rheumatologist or nephrologist has advised me. I know she just does not know how to handle my issues. Consequently, I have many people who care about me, but at the same time, they all depend on me to know what is going on and what I need. Sometimes that is scary because I wonder who will be there for me if I end up in the hospital and unable to make decisions for myself at some point.

Q: What would you tell a newly diagnosed person regarding the importance of having a support system?

A: Again, find someone who understands the disease as best as someone can. Then to the degree you are able, educate those who are closest to you so they have an idea of what you need. Be patient, understanding that things that you have to think about every day will not come so easily to those who do not feel what you feel. It does not mean they do not care. It is all too easy to associate everything with lupus, but try not to let lupus define who you are. It is a disease you have to live with but it is not who you are.

Q: Describe the positives in life even after a lupus diagnosis. What is your perspective on how you can lead a productive life even with the disease?

A: Oh my goodness, never give up. No matter how bad it feels, someone always has it worse than I do. I am thankful for what I can do, and if it really matters, I will find a way to do it. If that means I walk when my knee hurts, I walk. If I need to stop eating chocolate or marinara sauce because I have developed food sensitivities, then I will find something else I like just as much, or I will reward myself with one of those things anyway, followed by a Benadryl tab. Every day is a blank canvas and it can be what I make it. I will not let any disease be the boss of me.

Q: How does faith play a role in your disease? What are your beliefs and how have they helped you get through not only the difficult diagnosis, but also everyday hiccups that occur with lupus?

A: I am sure it plays a strong part. My faith is a big part of who I am, so it obviously has a lot to do with how I face any confrontation. It is not a religious object I pick up when I need it; it is who I am. It is what I believe just like I believe my name.

Q: What role has nutrition, healthy living and exercise played in your life? Do you exercise or follow any specific eating habits? And, have you ever consulted with a nutritionist?

A: I strongly believe that nutrition has a huge part to play in all disease and infirmity. I believe we are foolish with our bodies, like trying to run a car by pouring Kool-Aid in the tank. The body is designed to run on certain amounts of nutrients and exercise, yet we persistently fill them with junk, withhold things they need and do not give them the required amount of exercise. Of course, they start to break down. I have known this from the time I was a child. I have not lived by it however, and now I see the breakdown and wish I had. It is not too late however. I have started on a regimen of Shaklee food supplements, am in the beginning stages of an exercise regimen, and fully intend to get back to a fully functional and healthy lifestyle.

Q: How would you finish the following sentence?

I am becoming a better person through this experience...

A: I am becoming a better person through this experience with lupus because it has forced me to face things and make serious changes in my priorities. Maybe it is facing my own mortality, or realizing that I do not control everything in my life. It is helping me to be grateful for things I otherwise took for granted. It makes it easier to say, "I'm going to quit work early today so I can spend some time with my granddaughter, or call my mom."

Q: If your character, your life, your dreams, etc., could be summed up in one quote or motto, what would it be and why does it mean so much to you?

A: "You know all of those things you've always wanted to do? You should do them." I realize I have been guilty of talking about things I would do one day. Too much talking, not enough doing.

"Your life is a result of the choices you make. If you do not like your life, start making different choices." I understand not everything in life is a choice. I sure would not choose to have lupus. But, I can choose what I do about it and whether or not I let it dictate everything else I do.

"As a man thinks in his heart, so is he." This is so true. If you think you cannot do something, you have already failed. But, if you truly believe you can, you will find a way.

Q: *Who are the most important people in your life and why?*

A: My family, because they are my family and I love them. My best friend, because he has known me at my worst and still loves me anyway.

Q: *What are your plans for the future, despite lupus, and how do you plan to achieve them?*

A: I do not think about having lupus any more than I think about having blue eyes. I do realize I have some special needs because of it, so I adjust. If the sun is too bright, I wear sunglasses. If lupus means I have food sensitivities, I adjust my diet. If lupus means I get tired faster, I get more rest. It is what it is, but it does not control me. I decide what I can and cannot do and what I will achieve.

I finished my Master's degree in 1998. I have always intended to go on to finish my PhD. First, I want to get my 401k firmly in place and find a retirement home near a lake once my youngest is firmly ensconced in college, which should happen about a year from now. I also want to get at least one of my novels published, so I schedule a bit of time each week to work on it. I hope to have that in the works by this time next year as well. I like both short and long-term goals. It is hard to hit a target you cannot see.

Q: Last, please finish the following sentence:
Receiving a diagnosis of lupus...

A: Receiving a diagnosis of lupus after a long illness and search for answers was like having a light turned on in a dark room. For many months, I truly feared I was dying but no one could tell me why or from what. By the time I got the diagnosis, I wished it had been something with a better prognosis but I still felt a huge amount of relief. It is hard to fight something you cannot see or define, but now that I know what I am dealing with, I have viable choices. In a way, I have become more of a participant and less of a spectator in my own life. I like that. My future is good.

CHAPTER 12

The Story of Kia Paynes-Gentry

West Palm Beach
35 Years of Age
Medical Receptionist

Q: Kia, how you were diagnosed with lupus? What was happening in your life during that period, what age were you, and what type of symptoms were you experiencing?

A: I was 26 years old and working as a medical biller when I was diagnosed. I was outgoing, energetic and looking forward to doing many more things in my life. I started feeling fatigued and then I developed a rash (which I would soon discover was the famous "butterfly" rash) on my face. I went for tests and my primary care physician confirmed my diagnosis as Systemic Lupus Erythematosus.

Q: How would you describe your initial reaction to the diagnosis? Were you somewhat expecting it or did it come as a shock to you?

A: I was shocked, scared, taken aback, and overwhelmed. I did not know anything about the disease. I felt as if I was just diagnosed as "dead!"

Q: How does your initial reaction to the diagnosis differ from your outlook on life today?

A: I do not view my diagnosis as a death sentence. I have researched and taught myself about lupus. I no longer live in fear, but with the hope that we will find a cure.

Q: What are some tangible lessons that you would like to share with a newly diagnosed person or someone who is struggling with the disease?

A: For a newly diagnosed person, I would suggest to them to learn their limits. Remember that your body has changed and you have to learn how it responds to things all over again. It will be hard at first, especially when you may have once been used to jumping up and going out the door. It is not going to be that simple anymore. However, it can be manageable in time... with patience. It will also help to have a strong support system, as those are useful on so many different levels.

Q: What has changed in your life because of the disease? Did you switch majors in college, perhaps quit your job and started a completely unrelated occupation, change your plans regarding having children, move to a different location, etc.?

A: Personally, I have changed because of the disease. I have learned to remove myself from stressful situations. I am more relaxed and easygoing. My occupation has changed as well.

Q: What have you learned about yourself and your character through the lupus diagnosis? Has it made you stronger, more aware of taking care of yourself, or more compassionate?

A: Having lupus has helped me realize that life is too short. I am not so quick to judge people and their endeavors. Lupus has shown me how much of a fighter I really am.

Q: Do you consider yourself a fighter? What are some of the major hurdles you have had to deal with in terms of the disease? Think back to a moment you were very ill - how did you get to where you are now?

A: If I was unaware of my strength to fight before lupus, I was quickly taught. It was not even the numerous hospital stays from 2004 - 2006 (with severe seizures and high fevers) that brought me to that realization. It was in the year 2007, when I found out I was pregnant. As if hearing many doctors advise me that they would not take me on as a patient if I continue with the pregnancy was not bad enough, they also felt it would be dangerous to my life and they would have to choose whose life to save. My reality check came when I was hospitalized during my pregnancy due to a pulmonary embolism. This incident taught me how strong I truly was. My reward was looking into my healthy baby boy's face after he was born.

Q: Kia, tell me about your support system. Also, what would you tell a newly diagnosed person regarding the importance of having a support system?

A: My support system consists of good friends, my husband, kids, my doctors and most of all, my awesome God. A strong support system is very important to have. This disease is swift and quiet. People cannot look at you and see you are sick. Your support system is comprised of the people who pick you up when you are down. They help you out when every piece of you hurts. No one is beyond support. Whether it is your church family, blood family, friends or a lupus group, it is imperative to be able to reach out to someone.

Q: How does faith play a role in your disease? What are your beliefs and how have they helped you get through not only the difficult diagnosis, but also everyday hiccups that occur with lupus?

A: There is no question that lupus is a difficult disease to deal with. However, I gave birth to my miracle child while battling this disease. I have also become closer to my Savior. Am I a perfect person? No, of course not. I am, however, a faithful believer. I know that my Lord will never leave me nor forsake me. I did not know it at the beginning of this journey, but I now know that I have not ever endured the full wrath of lupus on my own; I have been carried through this whole endeavor by my God!

Q: What role has nutrition, healthy living and exercise played in your life? Do you exercise or follow any specific eating habits? And, have you ever consulted with a nutritionist?

A: I do not follow a specific diet nor do I exercise. However, I find that I have fewer flares when I eat carefully. I say carefully because I am not the healthiest of people. I try not to eat too much fast food and I am not really into sweets. However, I do eat a lot of bread and I am big on pasta. So, I try to manage how I eat those things. I keep my weight as balanced as I can while being on prednisone. I do admit (from experience) that if I did diet and exercise, it would contribute tremendously to a flare free lifestyle.

Q: How would you finish the following sentence?
I am stronger with lupus...

A: I am stronger with lupus because I refuse to back down. Even with lupus, I have a full-time job, two kids, a husband and I am still going strong.

Q: If your character, your life, your dreams, etc., could be summed up in one quote or motto, what would it be and why does it mean so much to you?

A: My favorite quote is, "If He brought you to it, He will carry you through it." I live by this quote every day.

Q: Who are the most important people in your life and why?

A: My family, friends, and always my God. I cannot live without Him; He wakes me up and lays me down. I would not have my family and friends if He did not deem me worthy of their love and support.

Q: *What are your plans for the future, despite lupus, and how do you plan to achieve them?*

A: I plan to live my life with God first and singing my praises until He is ready for me to come home.

Q: *What are three tangible pieces of advice that you would offer to someone struggling with the disease?*

A: Become one with your new body and mind. Do not give in to lupus. Fight, pray and live!

Q: *Last, please finish the following sentence:*
Even though I was diagnosed with lupus...

A: Even though I was diagnosed with lupus, I am much stronger now with the disease than I ever was before the disease.

CHAPTER 13

The Story of Kim Green

Atlanta, Georgia
46 Years of Age
Disabled/Freelance Writer

Q: Kim, how you were diagnosed with lupus? What was going on in your life during that period, what age were you, and what type of symptoms were you experiencing?

A: I was 37 and experiencing knee pain, chest pain and total exhaustion and weakness. At the time, my husband and I had just adopted a newborn baby. We owned an incredibly stressful business that was much bigger than I ever imagined or wanted, and my husband was straying. It was a time that I felt incredibly powerless in this life that I had created, and realized that it did not feel right. The baby had come and we were thrilled with him, but I felt that the whole thing was overwhelming on some cellular level. Right before I was diagnosed, I suddenly came down with Bells Palsy and they thought I had a stroke. Everything went downhill from that moment on.

Q: How would you describe your initial reaction to the diagnosis? Were you somewhat expecting it or did it come as a shock to you?

A: I was shocked and afraid that I was going to die. I felt the urge to blame myself for past transgressions. I was just desperate to make sense of it all.

Q: How does your initial reaction to the diagnosis differ from your outlook on life today?

A: I have settled into this illness and I feel like I have a fairly good handle on it. Seeing so many other people thriving with lupus has inspired me to keep going no matter how weak or ill I feel.

Q: What are some tangible lessons that you would like to share with a newly diagnosed person or someone who is struggling with the disease?

A: I would suggest that they survey their emotional life. Clean out the clutter that surrounds them - old friends, old things, old clothes, and old habits. I would also suggest that they do something they have always wanted to do and would not or could not in the past. The biggest issue is how to get right with yourself; be selfish for once. Even if a person is bedridden, they need to be thinking and dream-building about what they will do when they feel better. Be courageous enough to be alone if you are in an unfulfilling relationship.

Q: What has changed in your life because of the disease? Did you switch majors in college, perhaps quit your job and started a completely unrelated occupation, change your plans regarding having children, move to a different location, etc.?

A: I left my marriage, left the state, changed my work and became a single parent in a different state without the presence of my son's father.

Q: What have you learned about yourself and your character through the lupus diagnosis? Has it made you stronger, more aware of taking care of yourself, or more compassionate?

A: I have written a novel that details these very issues (www.hallucinationthenovel.com). What I learned most is the only person I can rely on is myself. And, that is a powerful and startling truth.

Q: Do you consider yourself a fighter? What are some of the major hurdles you have had to deal with in terms of the disease? Think back to a moment you were very ill - how did you get to where you are now?

A: I have been lucky compared to others that I have met. I am a fighter, but I am acutely aware that there could be harder battles to come. My biggest health issue is my nephritis. It keeps me perpetually vigilant and worried. I have since changed my diet drastically and tried implementing holistic practices to deal with the overall inflammation in my body. My arthritis is the most discouraging thing because being challenged with my mobility really hurts my soul. Every day that I feel energetic and ambitious is a winning day! Those days that I do not feel that way, I rest. Those are the fighting days.

Q: Kim, tell me about your support system.

A: I have a loving partner who is very familiar with lupus because ironically her older sister has it. She supports me by helping me with things that are too exhausting for me, has a strong relationship with my son and takes him when I cannot do anymore. She encourages me a lot to stay on track with my exercise and my diet, etc... Additionally, I have some great family friends and surrogate "mother" figures who take care of me by loving me and also loving and caring for my son.

Q: What would you tell a newly diagnosed person regarding the importance of having a support system?

A: I would tell them to really think about who they trust with their new life as a chronically ill person. Disappointment caused by false friends can cause a setback. Be very careful who you choose to support you, and once you trust them, *let them help you.*

Q: Describe the positives in life even after a lupus diagnosis. What is your perspective on how you can lead a productive life even with the disease?

A: The positives in my life are that I can finally take care of myself without so much career pressure and environmental stress. Lupus has demanded me to do this. I do not feel bad saying no to things or people that I do not want around me. I have really created a safe space for myself, which is crucial to feeling well. I have also learned about food and that has made me much healthier overall.

Q: How does faith play a role in your disease? What are your beliefs and how have they helped you get through not only the difficult diagnosis, but also everyday hiccups that occur with lupus?

A: My faith has grown tremendously. When I first moved to Atlanta, I did not have a faith community. I just prayed a lot and then I became a Unitarian. Although that is not a fundamentalist faith, the kindness and support that I have been given has helped me with my lupus profoundly. Just feeling loved and supported has been healing. I have felt comfortable enough to reveal my disease after not being able to before. I am no longer ashamed of having lupus. That has been a big step for me. I embrace it because it makes me fragile and human and connected to the human race, thus strengthening me. I no longer dream of being "perfect." Being "me" is now perfect.

Q: What role has nutrition, healthy living and exercise played in your life? Do you exercise or follow any specific eating habits? And, have you ever consulted with a nutritionist?

A: I did Weight Watchers and lost 23 pounds. I was also a long-distance walker, which was great and empowering.

It was the most healthy I have felt with this disease. Now I am a vegan (with some fish), and although I am concerned sometimes about my chronic anemia, I know I feel better without meat, dairy or even sugar in my diet. I do think that the reduction of meat and dairy help with the inflammation and hopefully will help with the kidney inflammation. That is where prayer comes in, after I have done everything I was supposed to do. I also do Yoga at home in the mornings, but mainly to center myself and get myself calm. Stress I think is the main agitator for my disease. And, l have to work very hard to stay centered. I notice that fried foods have a terrible impact on me as well as too much starch. I struggle with wheat bread; I am also trying to be gluten-free, but gluten-free bread is dreadful!

Q: How would you finish the following sentences?
Even with lupus, my life is all I have dreamed of because...
This disease will not cause me to stumble because...

A: Even with lupus, my life is all I have dreamed of because I have had the precious time to write, reflect and be the artist that I have always dreamed I would be. I have become stronger through this disease because I am strong enough to love myself.

This disease will not cause me to stumble because I have learned the power of my gift as a writer and I give it back in many ways to inspire others to truth and to find their voice. That is my ministry.

Q: If your character, your life, your dreams, etc., could be summed up in one quote or motto, what would it be and why does it mean so much to you?

A: "If nothing changes, nothing changes." Believe it or not, I got that quote from Weight Watchers and it means so much to me. Change and flexibility are the things that have saved me. The ability to go with the flow is a huge change for my spirit. There are no longer wrongs or rights. It just matters how my heart feels. Change is the most positive thing you can do to thrive.

Q: Who are the most important people in your life and why?

A: My son is the most important person in my life. I lost my mother when I was 15 years old and so I am acutely aware of how I do not want to die and leave my son without me. Just his very presence keeps me alive, as well as his amazing love and spirit.

Q: What are your plans for the future, despite lupus, and how do you plan to achieve them?

A: I plan to stay consistent in my eating habits and my spiritual practices. I plan to stay consistent in my relationships, continue to love myself, and stay spiritually vigilant and aware of harmful people, places and influences. I plan to thrive as a writer and an author. I plan to advocate for this scary condition that has changed my life and blessed it at the same time.

Q: What are three tangible pieces of advice that you would offer to someone struggling with the disease?

A: I would ask them to step back and survey their life; what they want, what they have denied themselves and who in their life has been toxic and damaging to their spirit. Then I would suggest that they read up on healthy food and how the human body works. Then I would ask them to design a life that strengthens them emotionally, spiritually and physically. And, if that means losing some people, places or things along the way, I would ask them to be courageous. Love yourself! And, take care of *you*.

Q: Last, please finish the following sentence:
Even though I was diagnosed with lupus...

A: Even though I was diagnosed with lupus, I am a far better person than I would have ever been without it. Lupus grounded me and gave me wings to be a compelling example of the frailty of life.

CHAPTER 14

The Story of Patty Guidice

Fishkill, NY
62 Years of Age
Office Manager

Q: Patty, how you were diagnosed with lupus? What was happening in your life during that period, what age were you, and what type of symptoms were you experiencing?

A: When I was 16, I was diagnosed with German measles and had pain in my joints and a rash. After the measles cleared up, I was still not feeling well with low-grade fever, joint swelling and chronic fatigue. My mother took me back to our general practitioner and wanted to know what was wrong with me. He told my mother that he was looking for something called lupus but could not find it. He told her to take me to Columbia Presbyterian Hospital in Manhattan. The next day she had me on the subway going to the hospital. When we arrived, we were taken into a clinic setting (this was back in the 60's). They gave me an exam, took a lot of blood and told me to come back in two weeks. We went back and they did not know anything else but sent me to a different clinic. When we got there, they called my name and told my mother they wanted to see me alone. The doctor took me into a cubical and asked me who I had sex with. I told him no one and he insisted I had to tell him because I had syphilis and they needed to know who I had sex with. I went outside and called for my mother and I told the doctor to tell my mother what he said I had. She said that the test was wrong, which of course led to many other tests. The doctor also said it could be hereditary and wanted my parents to be tested. My dad also said that he was wrong.

Finally, after about six weeks of tests and waiting, the final test showed that I had a false positive RPR. That is one of the symptoms for Antiphospholipid Antibodies. I then made it to the Arthritis Clinic and was seen by Dr. Carmen Neu. I had a kidney biopsy at 17 years of age. They broke a blood vessel; I hemorrhaged and had to have my kidney removed. After that, I had a flare every two years that required hospitalization. At 27 years old, I had bilateral hip replacements. In 1987, I had my first kidney transplant, which my brother gave me. My new kidney and I just celebrated our 25th anniversary! One year after the kidney transplant, I had to have my left hip revised. Then in 2003, they found a pituitary tumor. In 2006, I had my gallbladder and part of my intestine removed. In 2007, I had the pituitary tumor removed. And, in 2009, I had a hip revision and my second kidney transplant in December of 2010.

Q: How would you describe your initial reaction to the diagnosis? Were you somewhat expecting it or did it come as a shock to you?

A: It took about three months before they gave me the diagnosis. I was relieved to know what I had. I was expecting it after what our doctor told us. I think I handled it well because I had great support.

Q: How does your initial reaction to the diagnosis differ from your outlook on life today?

A: I have to say in the beginning I was my worst enemy. I thought I could do anything I wanted and learned the hard way that I cannot. I believe I was the cause of my flares every two years because I was not taking good care of myself. When I finally realized I was in control, I started doing things right - getting enough sleep, eating well and asking for help when I needed it. I finally realized that I needed to take charge of my life and do what was best for me. I was very lucky and was able to work full-time all these years. I met my wonderful husband and he has been a huge support to me throughout the thirty years we have been married.

Q: What have you learned about yourself and your character through the lupus diagnosis? Has it made you stronger, more aware of taking care of yourself, or more compassionate?

A: I believe it has made me a stronger women and I have been told I have a great outlook on life by all of my friends. Lupus has made me see how strong of a person I am and that I can handle what is given to me.

Q: Do you consider yourself a fighter? What are some of the major hurdles you have had to deal with in terms of the disease? Think back to a moment you were very ill · how did you get to where you are now?

A: I consider myself a huge fighter. My boss always tells me she does not know how I handle these things as they come along. She says that I am one of the strongest people she knows. I have had multiple surgeries and have always had my parents with me to get me through. It was hard when I lost my dad, but when I lost my mom it was awful. She was my best friend, and was there with me every step of the way.

Q: Patty, tell me about your support system.

A: My support system consists/consisted of my parents, brothers and of course my husband, who has been through all of these things with me. A month before my first transplant my mother-in-law passed away and then a month later, I had a kidney transplant. My poor husband was beside himself after going through that loss and then having me in surgery.

Q: What would you tell a newly diagnosed person regarding the importance of having a support system?

A: I would tell them that it is imperative that you have a great support system. It does not always have to be family. I do not know what I would have done without some of my friends helping me through this.

Q: Describe the positives in life even after a lupus diagnosis. What is your perspective on how you can lead a productive life even with the disease?

A: You need to realize that you are in control and are the only person who can help keep your disease in check. You can lead a very productive and happy life when you have a good doctor and family and friends supporting you.

Q: How does faith play a role in your disease? What are your beliefs and how have they helped you get through not only the difficult diagnosis, but also everyday hiccups that occur with lupus?

A: I firmly believe that without my faith in God I would not be here today. He has been by my side through thick and thin, and always answers my prayers. You need to believe in something or someone to help you live your life.

Q: What role has nutrition, healthy living and exercise played in your life? Do you exercise or follow any specific eating habits? And, have you ever consulted with a nutritionist?

A: I believe that a healthy diet with good nutritional value is the best. I do not follow any specific diet or take anything if I am unsure what it will do to my system. I exercise by walking my dog every day. I know that walking helps me clear my head and relax, and of course my dog is a wonderful companion.

Q: How would you finish the following sentences?
Even with lupus, my life is all I have dreamed of because...
I have become stronger through this disease...

A: Even with lupus, my life is all I have dreamed of because I have met and married a wonderful man who loves me and my disease.

I have become stronger through this disease because I have learned how to live and cope with it.

Q: Who are the most important people in your life and why?

A: The most important people in my life now are my husband and a multitude of family and friends who are always there for me.

Q: What are your plans for the future, despite lupus, and how do you plan to achieve them?

A: Right now my plan for the future is working a few more years so I can retire and move to Florida where it is warm all the time, with my husband.

Q: What are three tangible pieces of advice that you would offer to someone struggling with the disease?

A: Always have faith to help you through the tough times. Try to keep a good outlook on life and keep a stiff upper lip. Make sure you find a doctor who you really like and listens to your symptoms and problems.

Q: Last, please finish the following sentence:
Even though I was diagnosed with lupus...

A: Even though I was diagnosed with lupus, I have lived a happy and healthy life because of faith and family and friends. So, I can continue to live the rest of my life hopefully in remission.

CHAPTER 15

Perspective Highlight - A Sister's Perspective

By Amy Kelly-Yalden
President and CEO
Lupus Foundation of America Southeast Florida Chapter

Lupus has been in my life since I was a teenager when my sister, Erin, was diagnosed after years of illnesses and hospital visits.

I was the big sister. We were just three years apart but to me, from the time my mom told me my sister was growing in her belly, I told everyone she was my baby. I will say in 37 years that has never changed. Erin and I were complete opposites. I was the social one and she was the quiet one. I loved girly things. She did not like my girly things, and boy, did my Barbie dolls pay for that. I loved sports; she liked Lifetime movies. She had the black car; I had the white car. I was the people pleaser. With her, you had to earn her trust and friendship. Even the way we saw our future was different. I was going to get married and have kids early and she was going to be the career woman. Our differences only made us closer.

From as far back as I can remember Erin, or as I called her "Ernie," was sick with something · from mono and kidney issues to strange cysts and high fevers with no explanation. It was not until she was 19 and a freshman in college did she finally get a diagnosis of lupus. I remember hearing the word and wondering what it was. There was not much information available outside of learning it was an autoimmune disorder and she would need to take medications. She also had Hashimoto's, so I thought it was along the same line. And we did what we always did, continue with life.

Erin was my roommate in college. We both worked. The only time Erin seemed to slow down was to take a nap. She loved naps since she was born. She won "Best Napper" in kindergarten. Now I know that is what her body required because of the lupus.

So, that dream I mentioned of her being the career woman and me being the young wife and mom...switch people. When Erin was 20, and as stubborn as ever, she insisted on getting a puppy. We had just bought a small townhouse together and I compromised and said we could get a small one. I come home and there she was with her new puppy Jake, a Rottweiler. Those big brown eyes (hers, not the dog's) looked at me and I said, "Fine." Months later that little puppy was nearing 50 pounds and apparently very hungry. We came home one day to discover he ate our brand new carpet. Erin agreed the place may be too small and we may be too busy for Jake. We vowed to find him a loving (and large) home. One of my employees, Mat, was interested and we scheduled time for him to come meet Jake. Mat pulled up and Erin walked out with me. Those two sat and stared at each other for a good three minutes before speaking. I watched them fall in love right then and there. They got engaged. Erin finished school and became an Exceptional Student Education Specialist and her three beautiful sons, Kallen, Dane and Connor, soon followed.

Erin made it all look so easy. She worked full-time in a high pressure and often emotional job for the school board. She did not just love her job, she became a tireless child advocate. She had three boys despite her doctors suggesting otherwise. She always felt best when pregnant but would have her worst flares after each birth. Nevertheless, she was made to be a mommy and lived for her boys. And with three boys, you can imagine how hectic life was. All three boys were avid sports lovers. If there was a ball, they wanted to kick it or throw it. She worked a full day and then would be at the sidelines for practices and games then dinner, homework, baths, bedtime stories, snuggles and bed. And, the next day it would happen all over again. In the midst of these hectic days, there were days or weeks spent in the hospital a few times a year. It became part of our normal life. The boys even made a game out of the hospital beds and their remote control. Erin was on chemotherapy and steroids for years. Eventually biologics and weekly infusions became part of her treatment regimen. She made it look easy. It was not easy.

On February 24, 2009, at the age of 34, I received a call that forever changed our lives. Erin had died in her sleep.

Lupus had attacked her heart and eventually her heart gave out. I cannot even begin to tell you what her death has done to all of our lives. So much has changed. More than you can imagine.

Despite our extremely close relationship and the other close relationships in her life, Erin describes in her journal feeling very alone and isolated with her disease. When she received infusions she was often surrounded by seniors receiving treatment for Rheumatoid Arthritis. She only knew one person with lupus...her high school friend's mother who died from lupus complications at the age of 40. Because of that Erin, would occasionally tell us she did not think she would be here long and it is why she insisted that the boys have more than just her and their dad as part of their regular everyday lives. Maybe it was denial or thinking she was an exception, but we never took her warning seriously. We thought, "Who dies from lupus?" No one told us that people do. No one educated us. There was no community. No walk. No seminar. No helpline. There was nothing.

Erin would want those living with this disease to not isolate themselves. She would want them to embrace the growing community, support one another, to not live in silence with lupus and to add their voice to make a difference. And, she would want those who know or love someone with lupus, to educate themselves. I mean to really educate themselves about the reality of this disease and how it affects the person they love.

Today, I want a lot in terms of education and awareness, and I want it now. I want healthcare professionals to educate themselves. I want all rheumatologists to be willing to take a lupus patient. I want ERs to not be a scary place for the person living with lupus. I want more than one or two doctors in an area with 35,000 lupus patients to take Medicaid. I want more resources. I want more education and awareness and an arsenal of treatments options until we can find a cure. I want no one to feel alone with lupus ever. I want to see those living with this disease have better health care and surveillance. That means regular heart checkups (echocardiograms and EKG's), kidney tests, etc. I want those who love someone with lupus to learn everything there is to know about this disease and expose themselves to others living with lupus and listen to their stories. And, I want this community to stand up and demand more.

If we do not educate the public, tell the truth about this disease, and come out to events and programs, who will care? Yes, people will say, "You don't look sick," but if we do not tell them the truth and come together as a community then no one will care to think otherwise. We do not question someone who has cancer. We have empathy automatically regardless if their disease is visible. We support them and help them. That is because the cancer community has stood up and spoken out. I beg this community to do the same so no one else's story ends like Erin's. I do not want another child to lose their parent, or another mother or father to lose their child. I do not want another sibling to lose their best friend. This is our work. We must all do it together.

I was the Co-Founder and Executive Director of one of the world's largest cancer organizations in the world for over a decade. When Erin died, I reached out to the Lupus Foundation of America and asked to help. The local chapter in Florida was struggling as most non-profits were after the economic recession hit. As a born and raised Floridian, and as someone knowing the awful reality of this disease, I decided this was a fight I wanted to be part of. In two years, we have gone from just a few hundred people at a Walk to End Lupus Now event to a few thousand. During every walk, I choke up and feel Erin's presence and know how different her life would have been if she could have stood by those who know what it is like to live with lupus and see the outpouring of support from those that love them.

1.5 million people have this disease in the United States. That is 1 in 185 people. No one should ever feel alone. And, no one has to if we all work together to solve this cruel and mysterious disease.

CHAPTER 16

The Story of Elijah Julian Samaroo

Tamarac, FL
17 Years of Age
Fashion & Web Designer

Q: Elijah, how you were diagnosed with lupus? What was happening in your life during that period, what age were you, and what type of symptoms were you experiencing?

A: In July of 2007, I was 12 years old, about to hit the big 13 in August and start a new middle school magnet program. I was living in Albany, Georgia at the time and I was an outdoorsy kind of kid, especially with all the woods and outdoor areas we lived around. I frequently would walk through the brush around the woods in my backyard and often times the temperature would easily hit around 100 degrees. As the days winded down from summer break I started to have a red "hive-like" rash appear on my face. My parents took notice and thought I had come into contact with some poison ivy. After two weeks of the rash not going away, I went to the doctors in Georgia who immediately thought it was some kind of staph infection.

I was treated with numerous antibiotics and still no action. I was born and raised in Florida and overall the healthcare was better there, in my opinion. My parents decided to move back to Florida to give me a better chance in diagnosing the problem. In between jobs, my father had no insurance to cover me, so each doctor's visit cost hundreds of dollars. After visiting a dermatologist, he immediately recognized it as the butterfly rash and referred us to a rheumatologist, who sure enough told me I had SLE Lupus. Prior to this, I had no knowledge of what I had and not being in Florida for a year, I was dying to go to the beach. I ended up scarring my face worse than it already was, meanwhile I was starting 7th grade at a new school.

Q: How would you describe your initial reaction to the diagnosis? Were you somewhat expecting it or did it come as a shock to you?

A: My initial reaction to my diagnosis was a state of panic and shock. I thought my whole life was coming to end and it was all crashing down so fast. First, I had a huge rash/scar on my face and I was told I could not go in the sun anymore, had to wear sunblock, long sleeves, and use a hat and an umbrella. I was young and afraid about how the world would accept me. I did not know what to expect and neither did my parents. They never knew or even heard of lupus and what it entailed.

Q: How does your initial reaction to the diagnosis differ from your outlook on life today?

A: I was young at the time of diagnosis and I did not really know about much in life. I had always been a healthy kid so it really threw me off guard. Now I have totally embraced having lupus. I have a few scares here and there from my body rejecting medication and what not, but for the most part, I take it day by day and keep strong.

Q: What are some tangible lessons that you would like to share with a newly diagnosed person or someone who is struggling with the disease?

A: My few lessons I have learned are stick to your meds, your doctors definitely know what they are talking about and they are doing it for your best interest. Get a lot of rest and do not try to overexert yourself, but do enough that you do not become lazy. Your body will let you know and you just have to listen to the signs. Look for support among other people with lupus; they always are so welcoming and warm and will answer questions you have. They can definitely relate more than a professional that just studies lupus. Lastly, attitude is a major key to making it through the day. If your attitude is down and you are under stress, your body will reflect that and your lupus will flare up. You have to remain positive and be at ease from stress. It will not stop all of your symptoms, but it will definitely make them lighter on you.

Q: What has changed in your life because of the disease? Did you switch majors in college, perhaps quit your job and started a completely unrelated occupation, change your plans regarding having children, move to a different location, etc.?

A: Lupus affected my high school and middle school career because I missed half of my middle school years, and in high school, I started off home schooled. I tried going back to high school but had to be home schooled again in 10th grade. By 11th grade, I chose to drop out and get my GED, which actually was one of the best decisions I had made. I now do Web and Fashion Design and have full time to work and focus on it. In addition, I still have time to choose if I want to go to college or not.

Q: What have you learned about yourself and your character through the lupus diagnosis? Has it made you stronger, more aware of taking care of yourself, or more compassionate?

A: Lupus definitely has made me a stronger person. I get shots and do not even flinch. I am told I need an operation and I take it super easy. I am not worried that I will not make it through something. It also has made me realize that I have to take better care of myself and watch what I eat and do on a daily basis.

Q: Do you consider yourself a fighter? What are some of the major hurdles you have had to deal with in terms of the disease? Think back to a moment you were very ill · how did you get to where you are now?

A: I consider myself a fighter after all I have been through from being a rare case to overcoming many obstacles that have been thrown at me. I have gone through numerous operations, like biopsies and open-heart surgery, dialysis, chemotherapy and tests up the wazoo. I would say the hardest time for me was when I had open-heart surgery. I was a victim of anesthesia awareness and heard the entire surgery and post-surgery, where they had to intubate me and try to wake me up using various methods. Getting through that was a real test of strength and faith. I could not have done it without my family and God.

Q: Elijah, tell me about your support system.

A: My support system is comprised of my friends and family. Through thick and thin, they are always checking on me periodically and checking how I feel sometimes. I get annoyed sometimes but it is all love. My friends always find a way to make me crack a smile even in the toughest of times. Jokes from family and friends with their food definitely kept me going strong because I had a hard time eating hospital food, no offense to the cooks there.

Q: What would you tell a newly diagnosed person regarding the importance of having a support system?

A: Having one is important, whether it is your family and friends or other people with lupus. It is vital in respect to staying healthy and being strong. They can help you through anything and will keep your spirits high, which is necessary when you deal with all the complications of lupus.

Q: Describe the positives in life even after a lupus diagnosis. What is your perspective on how you can lead a productive life even with the disease?

A: Having lupus has given me the opportunity to meet and work with some people I see as role models and has given me new doors to walk through to lead me to a better life. I may have dropped out of school, which seems like such a bad thing, but I have never been happier. I work on what I love and I am able to support myself financially at such a young age.

Q: How does faith play a role in your disease? What are your beliefs and how have they helped you get through not only the difficult diagnosis, but also everyday hiccups that occur with lupus?

A: Faith plays a major role in my life. I pray as much as I can and when I was in the hospital for all those weeks, I would pray tremendously. My family and friends would come and pray with me. I am a Christian and we would have our local church pray for me as well as churches all around the world. That made me know I would make it through everything.

Q: What role has nutrition, healthy living and exercise played in your life? Do you exercise or follow any specific eating habits? And, have you ever consulted with a nutritionist?

A: Nutrition and some kind of exercise are vital. I try to eat as healthy and organic as possible, no sweets, no soda, and a lot of vegetables and fruits. I drink fruit juices and a lot of water to cleanse my kidneys; the key fruit juices I love are watermelon and pineapple juice. For some reason, they always make me feel better. I also try my best to stay away from fried foods and any kind of fast food. Eating that stuff makes me feel so sick and nobody wants to feel sick. Also, exercise as simple as walking the dog or walking around the block could make a drastic change. Participating in lupus walks are also a fun way to accomplish some exercise and be around people you can converse and connect with.

Q: How would you finish the following sentence? Lupus is...

A: Lupus is something I have, not something that has me. My life has been such an amazing experience even through it all and I would not change it for the world.

Q: If your character, your life, your dreams, etc., could be summed up in one quote or motto, what would it be and why does it mean so much to you?

A: "I am on the pursuit of awesomeness: excellence is the bare minimum." This is a quote by Kanye West that I like to live my life by. I try to make the most of life and be all I can be. I try to be happy and be fun. I have met many people who are consumed by lupus and I tell them they have to change and be happy about life, about the fact that we are still living and breathing. In the past few years, I have changed my whole attitude and if I were to describe my life with one word, it would be "awesome."

Q: Who are the most important people in your life and why?

A: My parents are definitely the most important people in my life. They always look out for me and not because they have to, but because they love me and want the best for me. I would not change them or adjust them in any way - they are perfect just the way they are. They would sleep together on a one-person cot in the hospital and be there at all times to get me whatever I wanted or needed. I could never repay them for that.

Q: What are your plans for the future, despite lupus, and how do you plan to achieve them?

A: My goal for the future is to take my current businesses to the next level and be more self-sufficient. I also want to find someone who understands me and makes me happy, create a family and teach them all I have learned in my life.

Q: What are three tangible pieces of advice that you would offer to someone struggling with the disease?

A: Surround yourself with positive people; they are your backbone. Do what you love to do, try to be the best at it and do not let your disease stop you by any means. Lastly, you must live your life; sometimes it feels like the lupus controls you but you cannot let it. Enjoy family and the small things, like rain or the air you breathe.

Q: Last, please finish the following sentence:
Even though I was diagnosed with lupus...

A: Even though I was diagnosed with lupus, I will never let it consume me or scare me like when I was first diagnosed. I will continue to fight harder and be stronger day by day and spread the love I have been shown.

CHAPTER 17

The Story of Jody Ortiz

Oklahoma City
44 Years of Age
Ghostwriter

Q: Jody, how you were diagnosed with lupus? What was happening in your life during that period, what age were you, and what type of symptoms were you experiencing?

A: I was diagnosed in 2003. I had just been married to my current husband for one year when my symptoms took over my life. At the time, I was a successful sales director with a cosmetics company. I had made it to the top 2% of the company within six months and I enjoyed what I did. I also was a Girl Scout leader, volunteered for St. Vincent de Paul Society, and I drove for Meals on Wheels. When I tried to donate blood at my church's blood drive, I got sick and my hands tingled and fell asleep. The technician advised me to see a doctor because she said that something must be wrong with me and that my blood would not be useable. I took her advice and went to the doctor. I was diagnosed with several things, including Sjogren's. My life was over as I knew it.

Q: How would you describe your initial reaction to the diagnosis? Were you somewhat expecting it or did it come as a shock to you?

A: My grandma had been diagnosed with lupus and almost died from it. Naturally, I was afraid of the diagnosis. I quit all of my volunteer activities and gave up my sales unit. I thought my life was over and that there was nothing more for me to do but to focus on my health. I even tried to file for Social Security.

Q: How does your initial reaction to the diagnosis differ from your outlook on life today?

A: My initial reaction was that it was the end of my world. Today, I love my life even more than before my diagnosis.

Q: What are some tangible lessons that you would like to share with a newly diagnosed person or someone who is struggling with the disease?

A: When I was first diagnosed, I was a super volunteer. It was hard for me to cut back, but I did and I feel better today. I took Plaquenil and medications that made me gain thirty pounds and lose part of my eyesight; I focused on the pain and the symptoms. Throughout the years, I have learned that my diagnosis does not define me. I do not take any lupus related medications today and I have learned to adjust my activities to fit my body's limits. I no longer have pain.

Q: What has changed in your life because of the disease? Did you switch majors in college, perhaps quit your job and started a completely unrelated occupation, change your plans regarding having children, move to a different location, etc.?

A: Since I gave up my sales unit and I did not have the strength to keep up with parties and meetings, I tried to file for Social Security and was denied. I then realized that as long as my mind worked, so could I. The doctors had me on pain medicine and anti-depressants and I had no idea what was going on half the time. I even left my house for an hour and a half with chicken cooking on the stove. When I arrived home, the house was filled with smoke and the chicken was black. That was a real turning point for me. I knew I had to get off the medication and reclaim my life. I figured out what made me sick and I just stopped doing those activities. I also started writing books for clients and set up my office so that I could write comfortably with a recliner and a wireless keyboard. It had been my dream to be a CPA, but instead, I became a writer. I was featured in our state's newspaper and did a news interview about my business and the fact that I switched from numbers to words. I found more success in my new career.

Q: What have you learned about yourself and your character through the lupus diagnosis? Has it made you stronger, more aware of taking care of yourself, or more compassionate?

A: I have become in tune with my body and I know what I can and cannot do. Before, I would work myself until I dropped and I went to the doctor every time I got sick. Now, I find natural ways of healing when I am ill and I stay within my physical limits.

Q: Do you consider yourself a fighter? What are some of the major hurdles you have had to deal with in terms of the disease? Think back to a moment you were very ill · how did you get to where you are now?

A: I learned how to fight for my life when I was turned down by Social Security and I almost burned down my home. I decided that I was in control and I have fought for everything since then.

Q: Jody, tell me about your support system.

A: My husband boxes for a hobby and he is from Mexico. That means that he is in great health and he believes in natural medicine. He has been a great support in helping me figure out how to live happily without the pain and feeling of worthlessness that came with my diagnosis. My daughter is in college and she was diagnosed with lupus when she was in the fourth grade. She has always struggled with her health and like me, she has learned to take care of herself. She understands what I go through and offers to help whenever I need it. We take care of each other and are able to sympathize.

Q: What would you tell a newly diagnosed person regarding the importance of having a support system?

A: Without a support system, you might end up depressed like I was. It makes life easier when you know that you have someone who understands what you are facing and who will help you.

Q: Describe the positives in life even after a lupus diagnosis. What is your perspective on how you can lead a productive life even with the disease?

A: My life has actually improved. I slowed down long enough to evaluate what I was doing with my life and I made some changes for the better. I believe that God does not make mistakes and He wanted me to suffer for a reason; I was going in the wrong direction. Now, I truly appreciate my life and feel even more fulfilled.

Q: How does faith play a role in your disease? What are your beliefs and how have they helped you get through not only the difficult diagnosis, but also everyday hiccups that occur with lupus?

A: Faith has played a big role. Because I know that God gives us challenges for a reason, I am able to focus on what is in store for me as His plan versus my disease.

Q: What role has nutrition, healthy living and exercise played in your life? Do you exercise or follow any specific eating habits? And, have you ever consulted with a nutritionist?

A: Exercise helps a lot. I now have a home gym with a treadmill, elliptical, and weight bench. When I exercise regularly, I feel a lot better. I am stronger and have more energy. I also eat much healthier. Fast food makes me ill, so I stay away from too many processed foods. I ate vegetarian and tried green smoothies for a couple of years but I ended up gaining weight, which made the arthritis even worse. Now, I make most of my food from scratch and I eat a balanced diet. I do not exercise as much as I should, but I am working on it.

Q: How would you finish the following sentence?
My life is better since my diagnosis because...

A: My life is better since my diagnosis because I found a talent I did not realize I had in writing.

I have beat this disease and I will continue to fight it because I am strong.

Q: If your character, your life, your dreams, etc., could be summed up in one quote or motto, what would it be and why does it mean so much to you?

A: My life's quote is "Carpe Diem," which means, "seize the day." That is how I live.

Q: Who are the most important people in your life and why?

A: The most important people in my life are my husband and daughter. I would not have been able to thrive without them and their support.

Q: What are your plans for the future, despite lupus, and how do you plan to achieve them?

A: I have now authored two books of my own and I plan to write several more. I have written over one hundred books for clients and I hope to someday reach the two hundred mark.

Q: What are three tangible pieces of advice that you would offer to someone struggling with the disease?

A: Your life is what you make of it. If you focus on the pain, you will feel pain. If you focus on the fact that you are alive and that you still have goals that you want to achieve, those will become your focus. Reach for those goals.

Q: Last, please finish the following sentence:
Even though I was diagnosed with lupus...

A: Even though I was diagnosed with lupus, I was able to defy the doctors and the specialists and create a life that is exactly what I want it to be.

CHAPTER 18

The Story of Jessica Goldman Foung

30 Years of Age
Freelance Food and Health Writer
Founder of www.SodiumGirl.com Author

Q: Jessica, how you were diagnosed with lupus? What was going on in your life during that period, what age were you, and what type of symptoms were you experiencing?

A: When I was thirteen, I arrived home from ballet class with swollen joints. As I come from a long line of autoimmune diseases on my mother's side, the swollen red nubs on my knuckles did not go unnoticed. Neither did the fact that my tonsils were a strange shade of grey; a discovery we made later that evening. Off I went to my first rheumatologist appointment, diagnosed with "potential" JRA, as my blood tests did not include any conclusive results. But, the symptoms were hard to ignore.

Believe it or not, though, this is hardly the start of my story. With my mother as my greatest role model, I learned to deal with chronic pain and fatigue without medication. I built quite a high tolerance to feeling "uncomfortable." And, I chose to keep the constant flurry of medical conditions ·

bloated stomach, rashes, migraines, blurry eyes · to myself. I just figured this was part of the disease. This was life; time to keep moving.

That is (luckily) when my body decided to speak up. At this point, the teenage ballerina at the beginning of our story was now a newly turned 21-year-old college student, studying abroad in Florence. I was feeling horrible, worn out and overwhelmed by a physical and emotional pain I was incapable of putting into words. Just in time, I arrived back home to California, ready to return to Stanford University for the winter quarter of my junior year. After a good night's rest, of course. However, like I said, my body had different plans. And, the evening before I returned to school, I looked in the mirror to see the Michelin Man staring back. I had an extreme amount of water weight on me and within a matter of days, a series of grand mal seizures landed me in the hospital. Suddenly, years of the unknown were revealed · I had Lupus. It was attacking my kidneys and my brain. And, I would not be moving back into my college dorm.

Q: How would you describe your initial reaction to the diagnosis? Were you somewhat expecting it or did it come as a shock to you?

A: In many ways I think we · my family, friends, doctors, and myself · were all shocked. Especially since, looking back at photos, the signs of the butterfly rash were very clear, from the rosy flush to the foggy eyes and brain. Those first few days, I was also fighting for my life. All my organs were under duress and it took everything and the kitchen sink to get me stabilized. So, while I was mostly in and out of a haze of drugs, I can only imagine the kind of shock felt by my parents.

In other ways, though, I was really ready for this battle and life with lupus. I had been having dreams for months before my rather dramatic diagnosis that I had cancer. I would gather loved ones and advise them that our fight would be one filled with giggles and shaved heads. I made friends with the men and woman who pushed my gurney. And, I cried every time I woke from these visions. When the reality actually hit, I was prepared. I knew exactly how I wanted to approach my diagnosis.

Q: How does your initial reaction to the diagnosis differ from your outlook on life today?

A: During my initial diagnosis, I was in survival mode. Man, it sure is a lot easier to live in the moment when you are in survival mode. Putting health and rest first on the priority list comes quite naturally. Pairing down activities to the essentials seems obvious. And, just waking up every morning is an accomplishment to celebrate.

The hardest part of the journey, though, came once I made it out of the hospital and started going back to school. Through great medicine, wonderful family and friends, and an enormous amount of support, I became stronger and healthier and miraculously, my kidneys started to work again. I had been given a gift—a chance to reenter the world. But, it was in this moment, when I started to recover, that the true uphill challenge began. Because I had survived, my toughest battle was not the one for my life, but trying to reclaim my life as it once was.

Q: What are some tangible lessons that you would like to share with a newly diagnosed person or someone who is struggling with the disease?

A: A portion of this answer is taken from an article I wrote for Crazysexylife.com. Someone long ago once said to me, when your life has changed, change your life. Considering how frequently I offer this advice, it would seem that I, myself, follow it loyally. But, the truth is, it has taken me almost a decade to actually put that advice into practice.

A few years ago, I left my full-time desk job—complete with mid-level management title, consistent paycheck, and fancy business cards—to confront the realities of my autoimmune disease and give myself a healthier, stress-free lifestyle. My new path as a freelance writer affords me the time and flexibility to see my doctors, pick up medication, and stay strong. But, I didn't get to this point easily or quickly. And, I spent many years trying to live beyond the realities of my disease.

When I was in survivor mode, the goal was clear: live. Nothing else mattered, and the simple act of sitting up in the morning, eating breakfast, and breathing were accomplishments. Once I survived, the goals of "real life" quickly seeped back in: graduate from college, hold a full-time job, save the world (and not just yourself).

It turns out that when your life has actually changed, the last thing you want to do is to diverge any further from your concept of normalcy. You would like to get back to it as soon as possible.

So, I got that desk job and I worked long hours like everyone else. I thought I had been maintaining a delicate balance of career, social life, and chronic illness. But, the reality was that the scales were greatly tipped and my health had become my last priority. Not only was there no time for doctors' appointments, the mere act of scheduling them was overwhelming. Everything—from my schedule to the fact that I sat in a chair for ten hours a day—was counter to what my body needed. Finally, five years post-diagnosis, I realized if I wanted to live a long and healthy life, I needed to make a drastic change. So, I did.

Today, I finally use those words that I have passed on to so many others. Since my life is now about my health, my health became the muse of my career. I began to write a blog about the adventures of living on a no-sodium diet, documenting the tasks and cooking experiments that take up much of my time. The blog grew into more articles about wellness, and I quickly realized that the daily health chores that once seemed roadblocks to success had become my greatest assets. The myriad of doctor appointments and long stays in waiting rooms were no longer in the way of my work, but what fueled my creativity and my writing. I had a defined niche, endless amounts of material, and—most importantly—I was doing something that would not only benefit me, but also others on a similar journey.

I thought that by listening to the needs of my body, my achievements would be stunted; the results have been quite the opposite. I am now the best version of myself, with the energy and mental capacity to accomplish more than I ever could before. Once I stopped trying to be ordinary, I could begin to approach my illness, my career, and, ultimately, my life by seeking the extraordinary.

Q: What has changed in your life because of the disease? Did you switch majors in college, perhaps quit your job and started a completely unrelated occupation, change your plans regarding having children, move to a different location, etc.?

A: Everything about my life has become more awesome. I tell people all the time that I would never trade my condition for anything in the world as it gave me focus, purpose, and the permission to actually put myself first - isn't that ironic?

Today, I race in triathlons, I work full-time as a food and health writer (one who lives on a salt-free diet, nonetheless); I backpack and travel abroad; I have a cookbook coming out in 2013; I'm about to become a mother; and I am able to do all of this while balancing the daily surprises that come with lupus.

Q: What have you learned about yourself and your character through the lupus diagnosis? Has it made you stronger, more aware of taking care of yourself, or more compassionate?

A: I like myself a lot. Not in a vain way - trust me, I would love to fix my teeth and let's not even talk about underarm "flippy flappies." But, I feel like lupus forced me to channel my spirit. I am goofy, positive, and an oversharer by nature - pieces of me which I used to be a bit weary of at times. These are the traits that help me survive and that continue to motivate me every day.

They are also what help me connect with others, whether they have lupus or are just dealing with a no good, very bad day. I feel more grounded and like I learn something about myself or the world around me every day. And, I go to bed every night more aware, present, and grateful than I could have ever imagined.

Q: Do you consider yourself a fighter? What are some of the major hurdles you have had to deal with in terms of the disease? Think back to a moment you were very ill - how did you get to where you are now?

A: I think I am a fighter. But more importantly, I am a solver. My hardest moment of the past decade with lupus was when I was finally released from the hospital and allowed to do dialysis at home. I was attached to a machine 12 hours a day, I had my driver's license revoked, I only saw friends when they visited, and I was living with my parents. I was 21 years old, bald and sick, with a 12-inch tube coming out of my stomach. It was the only time I really felt depressed and down.

Instead of getting angry, my parents and I had a pow-wow. We explored which parts of my routine we could potentially change in order to keep my spirit strong, all while sticking to my new health requirements. And, by looping in my doctors and doing research, the solutions started pouring in.

We found out that I could switch to a different kind of dialysis that would free me from the machine (or outpatient centers) and enable me to do my exchanges every three hours, by hand. We set up a room at my college so that I could attend a class every few days and do my dialysis treatments, in this special room, before and after the lectures. My parents even agreed to drive me to the college at dinner-time (and – do not tell my physician · parties as well) for brief interludes of "normalcy" as long as I wore a medical mask and was surrounded by a circle of my friends. We also planted a garden. We found a woman willing to teach me restorative yoga for 15 minutes, once a week, in my bedroom. And, another man who volunteered to teach me short dance classes when I felt well enough. A good friend even moved into my house for the summer between our junior and senior year so I always had social time, even if I could not get out of bed.

Rather than fight the realities of my disease, we came up with solutions to fill my "happiness" cup where we could. It is a practice I continue to this day. And, these little moments of "normalcy" buoyed my spirit, which in turn, greatly benefited my recovery.

Q: What would you tell a newly diagnosed person regarding the importance of having a support system?

A: You are your best advocate. You are the leader of your medical team. And, in a very short time, you will know your body better than anyone else, with or without a medical degree.

As such, it is important that you participate in your health care as much as possible and do what you can, beyond the office, to stay healthy. Keep a journal so that your doctors have detailed accounts of your symptoms. Treat every appointment like a creative writing class and describe symptoms as fully as possible; do not be shy. Tell your doctors what you need from them in order to live the life you want to lead.

Is it easier for you to communicate via email? Do you need a plan if something happens over the weekend and you do not want to rush off to the ER? Is a pill, diagnosis, or treatment plan not feeling right? Then ask your medical team about it and figure out a way to stay healthy and strong while living a life you love. The more proactive you are - both with your symptoms and your situation - the better your doctors can help you.

Q: What role has nutrition, healthy living and exercise played in your life? Do you exercise or follow any specific eating habits? And, have you ever consulted with a nutritionist?

A: For me and my particular case of lupus, a healthy lifestyle and diet have helped me stay alive, strong, and full. I keep a very strict low-sodium, salt-free diet due to my lupus-related kidney failure. And. what was once a simple doctors' order has transformed to a love of cooking and now, an actual career in food. It is kind of unbelievable that a restriction lead to limitless possibilities and a profession I once only dreamed of.

Q: If your character, your life, your dreams, etc., could be summed up in one quote or motto, what would it be and why does it mean so much to you?

A: "When your life has changed, change your life."

Q: Who are the most important people in your life and why?

A: I have been blessed with a large community of people who support me in everything I do. My mother, my dad, my brother, my husband, and my in-laws. No one treats me as if I am broken. They let me push myself, they respect my need to be young and active and even make mistakes at times. Yet, they are all there if and when I fall.

I am also lucky to have two women in my life, my mother and my cousin, who both have RA. I have this amazing built-in support group who understands what my life is like better than anyone else in the world. I have found it essential to have people like this in my life, with whom I can vent, cry, laugh, and have coffee · whenever I need to.

Q: What are three tangible pieces of advice that you would offer to someone struggling with the disease?

A: Focus on what you can gain from lupus versus what you could lose. Pat yourself on the back, every day, and celebrate everything you do; because accomplishing something in the face of lupus is ten times more impressive than meeting those goals without it. Do not let lupus define you; but do not forget to let it inspire you.

Q: Last, please finish the following sentence:
Even though I was diagnosed with lupus...

A: Even though I was diagnosed with lupus, I am more active, more grateful, and more inspired than before.

CHAPTER 19

The Story of Jonathan A. Ramirez

New Orleans
27 Years of Age
Civil Engineer

Q: Jonathan, how you were diagnosed with lupus? What was happening in your life during that period, what age were you, and what type of symptoms were you experiencing?

A: On the eve of my 22nd birthday, I was scheduled to have six wisdom teeth removed. Not four but six, I had two additional teeth sitting horizontally along the top row of my teeth. I was a university student at the time and had grown accustomed to the strange occurrences preceding this date. In isolated events up to four years before my diagnosis, I walked around with mouth sores, joint pain, thinning hair and eyebrows and fatigue, to name the most memorable ones. The term "walked around" cannot be used loosely, because this alone was a well-crafted balancing act as my heels regularly felt like they were made of glass. I moved on though, with a spring in my step (a very unique one, I might add) and attributed all of these matters to the environment of the plight of the retail working engineering student. I grew accustomed to opening my bedroom door every morning by placing my wrists on the doorknob and sliding them opposite one another. Holding a toothbrush, now that was another story. It is funny how something so simple is secretly so methodically balanced and choreographed by the human hand.

With six wisdom teeth removed and a face that resembled an inflated air mattress, I proceeded to take the required follow-up medications. I found that Penicillin works great, when you are not allergic to it. I quickly found out I was allergic and was asked to provide some urine samples to access the damage I had incurred. When the protein levels in my urine leaped off the page, my physician asked if I had a family history of lupus.

Four blood vials later, I was on my way to see a rheumatologist, nephrologist, dermatologist, and an ophthalmologist.

Q: How would you describe your initial reaction to the diagnosis? Were you somewhat expecting it or did it come as a shock to you?

A: When I was asked if I had a family history of lupus, I confidently chuckled and said "No." I had no idea what lupus meant, but something about the tone of the word quickly foreshadowed a very heavy set of hours to follow. My physician was of American descent, but she could have easily been a samurai warrior. The speed and precision with which she delivered this message resembled a steel sword penetrating an undisturbed pond. I could feel the indentation I made in the chair that I sat in as I began to realize I was suddenly a little less "Superman" and now a little more "Clark Kent." I was in a pure state of disbelief. I believed every word I was told but I could not believe I was no longer invincible. I always took great pride in not needing any kind of vitamin, medication or prescription.

Orange containers with strange names always belonged to older individuals at foreign dining tables. I had never seen a prescription sheet; that day I walked away with five. I knew my life had been too good to be true. There had to be some sort of anchor I thought. I was in a state of skepticism and confusion over what life was supposed to be used for and why it decided to let me know that I too had an expiration date. With my head held high, I exited the doctor's office for the last time as a casual visitor.

I then sent a text message to my girlfriend and best friend, "Well it is something called lupus, guess I am just going to have to beat this". Fortunately for me, I did not know how serious the illness was at the time. The more I read into it, the more I began to worry about how this was going to impact my collegiate plans. I wanted nothing more from life at the time then to become a civil engineer. That night I sat as people once did at late night drive-in theaters. The eight-millimeter horror film that played in my car was not projected on a giant screen but rather on the dark side of my eyelids. I sat in my car outside my university listening to my favorite musician and took refuge by digging my face into my palms.

The months to come were filled with moments of pain, anguish, anger, motivation and at times silence. There are only so many ways one can try to convey to others what a non-injured swollen knee feels like or how your fingertips repeatedly feel like they are being caressed by needles. Sometimes I wanted the pain to be on one extreme or the other. Pain can be physically taxing when its intense, but when it is mild, just mild enough to allow you to function, but strong enough to remind you it is there, that is when I would mentally breakdown. Then I began to lose my voice, but not literally. I began to lose my desire to share with others how I felt. You know deep inside that those closest to you can only hear you complain so many times. Feelings of withdrawal were inevitable only because you begin to feel like a burden on those who are willing to lend an ear to listen or offer some time to spend in your presence.

Q: How does your initial reaction to the diagnosis differ from your outlook on life today?

A: A lot of my time is spent on reflection. Pensive is a word that I would use to describe the first three years following my official diagnosis. To this day, I sit perplexed at the current state of my health. Just like the pains I would feel during my initial flares, Lupus is absent enough to allow me to function very well but present enough to remind me that it is still there. I have made friends with this illness, friends that I dare not compare my physical hardships with. The severity of my flares' are a drop in the ocean compared to those of some of my friends. This embodies the outlook I have life today. For reasons I have yet to grasp, I can still function in many ways that others cannot. Accordingly, I have come to believe that this comes with a set of responsibilities. I must come to terms with my situation and aid others by raising awareness about this illness. That keeps me going. I keep living because I know others who wish their loved ones could also. Were it not for them, I would quietly exist in my tiny corner of the universe with no intention to share these words with anyone.

Q: What are some tangible lessons that you would like to share with a newly diagnosed person or someone who is struggling with the disease?

A: Although every diagnosis is unique, rest always seems to work like a charm. Gauge your tolerances to the requirements of your daily life and do not let them deter you from accomplishing anything. Make adjustments as necessary. I did not know why I repeatedly struggled in school with fatigue and pain so all I could do was try to work around it. Sure, the time-frame in which I completed my goals may have been reduced had I not been experiencing any hardships, but the results were always to my benefit.

Learn to ask for help. I was and still am very hesitant when it comes to this because I strongly believe that I can always fix "me," but every now and then people and resources around us serve to remind me that they are always with me in this fight. I may not always need a hand with something but I have always found that simply knowing that there is one there should I need it, strengthens me two-fold.

Diet...there may not be a "lupus miracle food" but I do know that certain foods make you feel certain ways. Choose a diet and foods that make you operate at your greatest capacity and every shortfall that you may encounter will be that much smaller. Every bit helps.

Q: What has changed in your life because of the disease? Did you switch majors in college, perhaps quit your job and started a completely unrelated occupation, change your plans regarding having children, move to a different location, etc.?

A: Fortunately I have been lucky enough to have stuck to my original plans without altering too many of life's everyday actions with the exception of a healthy diet and flat out exposure to the sun. I long debated which goals would have to be modified or possibly left behind all together. However, these thoughts only made me incredibly stubborn and I chose to continue with everything I ever wanted to do as long as I felt physically and mentally capable to do so.

Q: What have you learned about yourself and your character through the lupus diagnosis? Has it made you stronger, more aware of taking care of yourself, or more compassionate?

A: In hindsight, lupus has served to get me exactly where I want to be in life. Along the way it has opened doors that I could not begin to imagine could have been possible any other way. Before my diagnosis, I did not know that I could speak publicly, network, and pursue community projects that extended outside the lupus community. The fact that lupus presented the possibility of incurring any physical limitations at any given time only made me want to excel at everything while I still could.

For many years, I was enthralled by the Afro-Brazilian martial art known as Capoeira. If you have ever seen it, you might safely make the presumption that one should be in top physical condition to take part. For a long time, I thought I was not strong enough so I never gave it any thought. Then lupus came along and I said the arthritis would never allow me to do this and it would just be another huge disappointment. Finally, some years later it dawned on me that I was not getting any younger, and whatever I had was here to stay. I said to myself once again, "I refuse to let this illness dictate how I will live my life." A year later, following one of the most uplifting activities I have ever taken part in, I know no physical or mental boundaries outside of just the required time and practice it takes to learn the martial art. And, I am the happiest I've been in years because of it.

This has made me stronger of both mind and body. I now know that there is more to what we see with our two eyes, that I could never imagine what others walk around with on a daily basis. This made me more sympathetic, compassionate, and patient to all actions, events and human beings. I now feel taller and wiser because of these experiences.

Q: Jonathan, tell me about your support system.

A: My support system continues to evolve with what I find to be my need for that time in my life. When I was in college, it was easy to focus in terms of semesters with regular faces that worked on the same goal. The task then was to surround myself with those individuals and select a few who could acknowledge my condition and ignore it as well. By "ignore it," I would stress that this is by no means people who were not ready to vent when need be, but knew when to push for our shared goal and when to let me figure out how to clear whichever manifestation of a flare I was faced with that day. For example, I remember very well preparing for a physics final exam. My preparation did not include the standard methods for optimal performance on a test, which included constant review and practice problems leading up to the test. My unwelcomed preparation consisted of a sore neck and laptop keys imprinted on my forehead from the nap I took in the library hours before the exam. My friends knew when to hassle me for being lazy and when to stop because none of us were able to explain how I could require so much sleep the morning after a good night's rest.

The fact that many episodes similar to these could not be explained prior to my diagnosis served me in a positive sense. Since we did not know what it was, there was no reason to give up. I could not succumb to feelings of inferiority because mouth sores just came from "using too much mouthwash" and heel pain from "too much long distance running in worn out shoes."

My family provided support in the same way. Our lack of knowledge on the signs presenting themselves all around us allowed my family to put off the struggles as mere inconveniences that were part of a very active lifestyle. Be it an ignorant bliss as it may, when news on the diagnosis gave us something to blame, the approach was the same. They were always there to listen, but were also there to act as a giant mediator that could deflect whatever ill feelings I had toward lupus and rather convert them into ill feelings I had toward a situation... a situation that I could always overcome. The less they knew about the disease, the easier it was to not allow me to fuel this unknown mystery villain. Looking back now, it helps me better understand the "swift punch" delivery I received from my doctor when she told me my diagnosis. With no time to dwell on it, all I could do was act on it.

Q: Describe the positives in life even after a lupus diagnosis. What is your perspective on how you can lead a productive life even with the disease?

A: Lupus has been an excuse to get angry at myself for believing that I am incapable of accomplishing anything for any reason. Before I was diagnosed, it was easy to flow through life scared or afraid to be uncomfortable or expose any weakness, be it public speaking, pursuing career goals or even physical activities. Lupus always carried a gravity only replicated by imploding stars. I literally began to grow tired of all the attention I gave something I dreaded so much. Eventually, all I could do was cross my arms, tilt my head back and think, "Well now I really have nothing to lose." A grin would then sneak its way on to my face and I would dive headfirst into whatever I felt that I could not do because of my illness.

Writing about lupus got me my first scholarship (The Michael Barlin Scholarship) and it was a very generous one nonetheless. At the reception for this award, I was asked to say a few words as a sign of gratitude. Nothing rehearsed or scripted, I simply said how I felt. The great people in that room were moved and asked me to do the same a year later. This provided a unique paragraph to add to a cover letter for the job of my dreams. The scholarship was then a topic of great curiosity in the interview that followed this cover letter. Where did I get the courage to bring up something I feared could blacklist me in the corporate world forever? I still wonder to this day. I got the job. Since then I became a board member for the Lupus Foundation in my home state of Florida and have been asked to speak on multiple occasions at very nice locations. I have raised my eyes to magnificent sights in ballrooms and auditoriums each stemming from those all too familiar LED lights in hospitals.

These events were inspired by people in the lupus community that, for reasons unknown to me, chose to help others afflicted with something that has devastated their lives so much. My desire to repay these individuals has extended beyond the lupus community and I have attempted to do the same for teachers. Using the experiences and knowledge I have slowly gathered from our outreach efforts with lupus, it has allowed me to make strides in other fronts involving education and engineering.

As a fan of mathematics, I could not explain to you how so much positive has resulted from something so negative.

Q: What role has nutrition, healthy living and exercise played in your life? Do you exercise or follow any specific eating habits? And, have you ever consulted with a nutritionist?

A: Nutrition, healthy living and exercise have each played an immeasurable role in my health. I maintained an active lifestyle before, during and after my diagnosis and so it is difficult to say whether or not it plays a role. However, I can say that when I cannot take part in some form of exercise my body seems to dwell on weakness. It may all just be mental, but knowing that I am in peak physical form allows my mind to be very confident and convinces me that I am too strong to be phased by anything. Also, perception allows me to fool myself into attributing any strange pain or fatigue to a rigorous workout or training session I may have had that day. For instance, I would much rather believe that I am feeling tired from an intense leg workout the night before than to say to myself , "Great, my lupus is acting up again."

Q: If your character, your life, your dreams, etc., could be summed up in one quote or motto, what would it be and why does it mean so much to you?

A: "When one door closes... you jump out a window." This comedic approach embodies my entire outlook on lupus. I heard it during a speech given by an engineer at a conference after receiving a scholarship to attend. The opportunity presented itself right after my diagnosis. It was as if everything came together so that I could fly across the country and hear those words. It taught me that doors will close all the time, some may be shut with no warning, others more gradually. Why sit there and stare at a shut door as if it is your only way out? A little thought, creativity, and wit can render any situation to your advantage and the outcome may be the same, if not greater, than whatever you may have anticipated in the first place.

Q: Last, please finish the following sentence:
Even though I was diagnosed with lupus...

A: Even though I was diagnosed with lupus, I continue to believe that my disability has not been anything but enabling.

CHAPTER 20

The Story of Marisa Zeppieri-Caruana

35 Years of Age
New York & Florida
Author, freelance journalist and "foodie"

Q: Marisa, how you were diagnosed with lupus? What was going on in your life during that period, what age were you, and what type of symptoms were you experiencing?

A: My lupus diagnosis came a few weeks after I was in a horrible accident. Before I get into the details, I will say that I have had health issues since I was a little girl. Strange fevers, mouth sores, pain and feeling ill after being in the sun were common occurrences. We could not afford health insurance when I was younger, which meant I could not get specific tests, so my doctor at that time really did not know what to tell me or my mother. We knew something "wasn't right" but I would have to learn to live with it.

My accident happened on the night of April 22, 2001 in Fort Lauderdale. I was hit by a pick-up truck while walking to my car. The truck was speeding and the driver was under the influence of drugs and alcohol at the time. As I laid on the asphalt, unable to move, I knew my body was badly injured. All I kept thinking about was if I would see my family again. The next thing I knew, I woke up in a trauma hospital surrounded by a room of people – doctors, a surgeon, my mother, nurses, police and my friends (who were outside of the room peeking in through the glass). I kept hearing phrases like "broken ribs," "liver lacerations," "internal bleeding," "fractured pelvic bone," "head injury," etc. On top of all of those injuries, I had also fractured my wrist and elbow on my right side and had painful road rash.

Apparently, when my floater ribs broke, they lacerated my liver into four sections – and the internal bleeding it caused was quite bad. I honestly do not remember much about my hospital visit, except that I was on a morphine drip and could barely talk. After some time in the trauma unit, I was moved to a regular room and then a rehab. I had to learn how to slowly walk again with the assistance of a cane and walker, as putting any pressure on my liver could cause it to start bleeding again.

A few weeks after the accident, I had a minor stroke. The doctors were not sure if it had something to do with the head injury, but once I broke out in a rash and spiked a fever (within 24 hours), they decided to do further blood work. I was lucky in a sense; so much happened at once in terms of symptoms, when the blood work came back, I was swiftly given a diagnosis of SLE Lupus. The doctors felt the severe physical trauma caused by the accident brought my body to a weak enough state that allowed the lupus to run rampant.

This was a bittersweet time in my life. One on hand, I was thrilled that I was "given another chance" in terms of the accident. The trauma surgeon had explained to me how lucky I was – that most pedestrians never make it to the hospital. But, on the other hand, I was feeling terrible and now told that I had some strange disease that no one was really familiar with. My entire life changed within a few weeks. I went from an overactive, full-time college student, with a full-time job and enough energy for ten people, to fighting for my life after the accident, and being handed a shocking medical diagnosis. I had to quit school for one year to recuperate, lost my job, and was bed bound for long periods of time in order for my liver to heal. I did not know it then, but this event was about to alter my entire "life plan" and steer me in a different direction.

Q: How would you describe your initial reaction to the diagnosis? Were you somewhat expecting it or did it come as a shock to you?

A: My initial reaction was one of relief. All of my ailments as a child suddenly made sense. Once my mom and I familiarized ourselves with the symptoms of lupus, it was clear that I had been experiencing them for many years. Personally, I did not feel so "crazy" anymore in terms of having weird symptoms and feeling sick often. When I did not have an official diagnosis, I would sometimes be brushed off by medical personnel. They made me feel like my symptoms were "all in my head." But I know my body best, and I knew something was not right; the diagnosis confirmed all of this for me. I think the "shocking" part of the diagnosis was that it was given to me immediately after the accident. I was already having a hard time making sense of that event, and was now given something else to deal with on top of it.

Q: What are some tangible lessons that you would like to share with a newly diagnosed person or someone who is struggling with the disease?

A: First, get to intimately know your body. When my husband first suggested to me many years ago to start journaling, I thought it was a silly idea. But, over time I decided to try it. I bought a day calendar that was small enough to fit in my purse, but had large enough daily sections that I could write down details. I would write down what I ate, what meds I took, and what activities I did. I would also write down symptoms I was experiencing, such as mouth or nose sores, fatigue, fever, pain, chest pain, etc. Over time, I began to see my "trends." Knowing what activity, food, etc. brought out worse symptoms or a flare up became a useful tool for the future. Now I knew exactly what to avoid. So, journaling would be my first suggestion.

Educating yourself is another helpful tool. While your physician can offer some information, do not rely on him or her solely when it comes to lupus education. There are some terrific lupus organizations that have websites packed with helpful information. Read brochures, books, pamphlets, etc. and try to reach out to others who have the disease. I cannot tell you how much I learned about lupus from speaking to other patients.

Most importantly, do not feel ashamed, embarrassed or feel like you have to make excuses for yourself and how you are feeling. For a long time, I was embarrassed to tell people that I had lupus because hardly anyone knew what it was. I also had a horrible experience with a dentist who refused to treat me because I had mouth sores. He asked me if I had HIV in front of other office personnel and when I explained that I had lupus, he seemed to not believe me or understand. Then he asked me to see another dentist because he "did not feel comfortable." I felt like a leper.

Over the years, I also ran into people who would tell me I did not look sick, or that I was feeling bad because I was "not exercising enough" or I was "sleeping too much." Overtime, I realized these people were just poorly educated about what lupus was. These people actually helped me fuel my desire to educate those around me on the disease. I would tell other lupus patients that you do not need to defend yourself when people are making light of your diagnosis or treating you like an outcast. It is best to just walk away with your head high, and if the occasion ever arises, educate them on what they do not know.

Q: What has changed in your life because of the disease? Did you switch majors in college, perhaps quit your job and started a completely unrelated occupation, change your plans regarding having children, move to a different location, etc.?

A: As I mentioned earlier, my entire life changed. After completing a few years as a chemistry major in school, I had decided to begin the RN program. I was a good student, on the honor roll, and was working full-time when lupus derailed my plans. I believe the stress of nursing school and working caused my lupus to flare, and the next thing I knew, I was being hospitalized for a pulmonary embolism. My doctors warned me that my lupus was active, I was not allowing by body to rest, was about to go into a profession where I would be in constant contact with infectious germs and that I needed to "rethink" my plan. I was extremely stubborn and tried to finish the program. One day, my body said "no more." I was hospitalized and could barely move.

I was crushed; I had worked so hard in school and was excited about being an RN.

After another year of recuperating, and spending many hours in bed, I rekindled an old love of mine – writing. One day, during a time of frustration, I prayed to God that He would open a door, show me a sign...just do something that would help me in terms of having a career. I am a true "Type A" personality and it was killing me that I could not hold a full-time job or even be an active member of society. I wanted to be doing all of the things my friends were doing – getting married, having a career, and having children. Three days after that prayer, I received a phone call from an editor of our local newspaper. She had seen something I wrote and casually sent to a friend and asked if I would be interested in writing for the paper. And so, in an instant, my writing career began.

Q: What have you learned about yourself and your character through the lupus diagnosis? Has it made you stronger, more aware of taking care of yourself, or more compassionate?

A: I learned that I do not give up easily and I continue to fight, even when the odds are against me. I have also formed a close relationship with God. Although I have always believed in God, the accident really propelled me into seeking a closer relationship with Him. The accident made me realize how life can be taken from us in an instant, and how lucky I was to be alive. I felt that God obviously had a purpose for me to be here, and since my life was not taken in that accident, I was given more time to fulfill that purpose. I have also learned to be more thankful. I did not have an easy life growing up and I had a tendency to focus on the things I did not have. I think that is what fueled me in educating myself, in order to make a good living and be able to take care of myself. But, once everything was taken away from me after the accident, I started to become thankful for the little things in life. Most importantly, I was just thankful to be alive – that alone was enough.

Q: Do you consider yourself a fighter? What are some of the major hurdles you have had to deal with in terms of the disease? Think back to a moment you were very ill · how did you get to where you are now?

A: I feel silly using the term "fighter," but I will say I am a strong person – physically, emotionally and mentally. The accident and lupus diagnosis were two major hurdles, but there was a third that came many years later that truly tested me. I was recently married to my amazing husband. I had been going downhill, in terms of lupus symptoms, for quite some time. On our honeymoon, my grandmother – who practically raised me – was rushed to the hospital and later died. That was a tremendous loss for me. A few weeks later, I was diagnosed with a brain aneurysm…and within a few months, I went downhill to the point of becoming wheelchair bound. Things continued to get worse. I began to lose weight for no reason and was eventually 89 pounds. I could not feed or bathe myself, or even get out of bed. When my mother and husband took me to the hospital, the doctors basically said I would not be coming home. Needless to say, this was a very stressful time for a newlywed couple. We soon discovered that my illness was caused by Plaquenil toxicity - a rare occurrence. In my case, I had been on it for nine years, was on a very large dose, and my body just could not flush it out fast enough. I had jaundice, heart enlargement, low blood pressure and low potassium. I stopped eating and basically gave up.

The doctors and I decided I would go off the Plaquenil while in the hospital to see if I would begin to improve. Within a week, the jaundice cleared up, and within three weeks my heart was no longer enlarged. I was also able to sit up and feed myself. At my lowest point during this period, I had prayed to God that if my "mission" in life was complete, to please let me come home. God did act on that prayer request by letting me have more time…another chance. I realized, yet again, that it was not *His* time for me to come home.

Once I was stabilized, I never took the Plaquenil again. Between the help of my amazing mother and husband, a new food plan, six months of exercising to get me out of the wheelchair, and a little prednisone, I was back to my old self. The best part of my recovery was that I had to gain twenty pounds to get back to my normal weight – and that allowed me to eat just about anything I could get my hands on. My family does not call me the "cookie monster" for nothing!

Q: Marisa, tell me about your support system.

A: I am thankful to have an incredible support system. My husband is a saint for dealing with me and lupus on a daily basis. I was also lucky enough to be given the most patient and loving mother in the world. They have both nursed me back to health many times. My grandparents were also a huge support for me when they were alive.

I also have some incredibly understanding and compassionate friends. They have seen the good times and the bad, and have stood with me through all of it. Over the years, I have also met a great group of men and women who have lupus. These people are a tremendous help when I need to speak to someone who can relate to what I am going through.

Most of all, God has been my ultimate support. Over the last twelve years, I have come to know that I am never alone. Through this disease, and the hard times, I am still confident God has a plan for my life. I know He will use this disease for something good and reassures me of this through Romans 8:28, which states, *"And we know that*

God causes all things to work together for good to those who love God, to those who are called according to His purpose."

Q: *What would you tell a newly diagnosed person regarding the importance of having a support system?*

A: Having a support system is crucial in dealing with this disease. No one should have to deal with this disease alone, and no matter how strong you are, there will be times when this disease will test you to your limits. Those are the times you will want and need loving family and friends around. If your family members or friends are not supportive, reach out to a local support group, online forum, or lupus chapter. There is always someone out there who will help you through the difficult periods.

Q: *Describe the positives in life even after a lupus diagnosis. What is your perspective on how you can lead a productive life even with the disease?*

A: The positive is that you can still live with lupus! It may take some medication, and tweaking your lifestyle or career, but it is possible. I believe everyone has certain talents and gifts, and we are given them for a reason. I always had a love for writing but never thought I would use it for any specific purpose. Now, I turned that gift into a career.

Lupus can be worked around and you can make it fit into your life, rather than stopping your life and your plans to fit into lupus. It may be hard to remember this on the tough days, so write it down if you need to – Even with lupus, you are still in charge of your body, your life and your future.

Q: How does faith play a role in your disease? What are your beliefs and how have they helped you get through not only the difficult diagnosis, but also everyday hiccups that occur with lupus?

A: My faith has been a major source of strength for me. It helps me with my anxiety when I am facing a lupus flare or a sudden emergency room visit, and it keeps me grounded when I get ahead of myself. Before the accident and diagnosis, I was completely wrapped up in the world – what I looked like, what career I would have, how much money I would make, and how I was going to survive. I only depended on and worried about myself. It was a self-centered way to live. I was young and very naïve about life.

After my own body failed me so to speak, I realized I cannot do everything in my own strength. And, knowing that I was lucky enough just to survive the accident, I stopped and finally looked at the bigger picture. *Why am I still alive? Why was I spared? What am I supposed to do with my life?* The accident stopped me in my tracks and veered me on a completely different life course. Once I began a closer relationship with God, I realized that all of the things that have happened to me have happened for a reason. I have no doubt that God has a special plan for each of us. He has helped me take two things I love – writing and helping people – and turn it into a fulfilling career and lifestyle.

Q: What role has nutrition, healthy living and exercise played in your life? Do you exercise or follow any specific eating habits? And, have you ever consulted with a nutritionist?

A: Nutrition is one of the most important aspects of my life in dealing with lupus. I have been able to control most of my symptoms with a very small dose of prednisone and a complete change in diet. After journaling for many years, I realized what foods made me feel worse. I now follow a mostly raw, vegetarian diet that includes juicing vegetables twice a day. This isn't to say that I avoid meat completely. I love chicken, and once in a while, I will treat myself to a piece. Also, like I previously mentioned, I am a cookie monster. So, I learned how to make cookies with a variety of flours and healthy ingredients. I have also spent about two years researching anti-inflammatory and Mediterranean diets and I now try to incorporate that into my daily menu. When I strictly follow this way of eating, I feel my best. Holidays can be tricky though, and after a day or two of eating any processed food, I immediately feel worse.

In terms of supplements, I take many that were recommended to me through nutritional counselors. In addition to juicing, I use a supplement called Rockin' Wellness, which helps immensely with my energy and I use a water-alkalizing machine that was gifted to me through LifeIonizers. I have tried many things over the past twelve years, but I now know what works for me and try to stick with those on a daily basis.

I would recommend any lupus patient to take a good look at the food they are eating and consider looking into healthy alternatives. Although there is no specific diet for lupus, from personal experience, I can say that diet has made all the difference. Exercise, while it has been difficult for me, also is a huge help in dealing with the disease. I love to swim and practice yoga. They are low impact and can really strengthen the entire body.

Q: How would you finish the following sentence?
Even with Lupus, my life is all I have dreamed of because...

A: Even with lupus, my life is all I have dreamed of because I have not allowed the disease to break my spirit and stop me from living. I have a wonderful husband and family, and even though my original life plans have been changed, the outcome has been more amazing than anything I could have ever imagined.

Q: Who are the most important people in your life and why?

A: My husband, Mickey, and my amazing mother. I could never repay them for all of the support and love they have shown me. My husband has been an incredible help because he always sees the best in every situation, always speaks the positives when I get hung up on the negatives, and he is forever the optimist. I am so lucky to have someone with this attitude in my life. Also, my brother and his wife have been a great support, as well as my friends.

My rescue dog Bogey has also brought me immense joy. We rescued him after reading that he had a major heart defect and was going to be put to sleep. He is completely unaware of his "disease" and lives every day to the fullest. He has shown me that life is meant to be lived, despite having a physical condition that impairs you. Some of my physicians have also been very important to me – they are caring and understanding of the disease and how it affects someone on a daily basis.

Q: What are your plans for the future, despite lupus, and how do you plan to achieve them?

A: Honestly, I just want to enjoy my life. Sometimes, I feel like I am on a shorter time period than everyone else in terms of achieving things in life and making a difference. That feeling propels me to get many things accomplished...quickly. It also has the ability to stress my body out and put me in a flare, so I have to be careful not to cross that line. I have outlines for five more books right now, and as my health allows, I plan to complete what I can. I am not in as much of a rush as I used to be. I know God has a plan for my future and things that I need to accomplish while I am here; my plan is to learn what those things are and to do them to the best of my ability.

Q: What are three tangible pieces of advice that you would offer to someone struggling with the disease?

A: Put yourself first – when you are tired, rest. When you feel like you might be going into a flare, see your doctor, take your medication and listen to your body. Take your diet and exercise into consideration.

Also, make peace with the disease — whether it is through your faith or with the help of a counselor who deals with chronic illness. Once you no longer see lupus as a disability, an entirely new world will open up for you. In addition, find support for the difficult times — whether through friends, family or a support group. If you cannot leave the house, consider an online support group. And, if you do get connected with a support group, try to find one that focuses on the positive.

Q: Last, please finish the following sentence:
Even though I was diagnosed with lupus...

A: Even though I was diagnosed with lupus, I believe I was created with a special purpose, plan and talents. Although I have no idea how much time I have, I hope to use these talents to help as many people as possible. I focus now on what legacy I can leave behind. I hope my books, including this one, can help lupus patients for many years to come. Even though I have lupus, I will never give up.

CHAPTER 21

Perspective Highlight – A Best Friend's Perspective

By Karla McLaren

I had met her on a few other occasions. She was the wife of my husband's oldest and dearest friend. I was visiting her in the hospital that day. As I walked into her hospital room, I tried to act as if her appearance had not left me aghast. As I tried to keep my composure, I hoped that she could not read the shock that was written all over my face. Her frail body had withered away to nothing. She was emaciated. Her complexion had turned yellow and her eyes were sunken and showed little sign of strength. Her mother gave my husband and I a run-down of the list of symptoms and medications that they had her on. To be honest, I did not understand most of it, but what I did pick up was that she was dying. She had lupus. We prayed with them, stayed a little while longer and left when we could tell that she wanted to get some rest.

By the grace of God, Marisa survived that horrendous ordeal, and several months later she and I would be reunited. This time, we would be drawn to one another by our mutual love of humor, food, faith and just about everything else that you can imagine. She just *got* me, you know? Some might call it a kindred spirit. We could talk openly and honestly about almost anything. There was never any judgment. We could literally talk on the phone for hours about everything from rising tensions in Syria to the latest flavor of M&Ms. One topic that frequently came up was lupus. I will be honest, before I met her, I had never heard of lupus. Over the next several years however, it would become proverbial.

One of the first lessons that I learned was flexibility. Marisa was at the mercy of lupus, and in turn so was I. At least, that was the case whenever we made plans. I could always hear the excitement in her voice any time that I suggested something fun for us to do for the weekend. We would spend the week planning what we were going to wear or ironing out details, but in the back of our minds we both knew that if there was a flare-up or a fever, we would have to take a rain check. I hated to see the disappointment in her face. Unfortunately, I saw it all too often. In spite of our plans going south though, we always managed to have fun. Hanging out at her place with delicious takeout, a great (or really stupid) movie, and good friends became a weekly routine. It was a routine that emphasized appreciating and enjoying the people in our lives.

The second lesson that I learned was that sick does not mean helpless and hopeless. In spite of the daily challenges that Marisa faces, she works harder than anyone I know. In the face of fever, pain, arrhythmias, and fatigue, she still logs an impressive number of hours a week. Why? Because it is part of her contribution to the world. I am sure that it would be a lot easier for her to stop working and focus on her illness, but then you are living for something that will not give you anything back. Instead, she chooses to focus on her gifts. The effects of those gifts will be felt long after we are gone. That is what she focuses on when she feels like she simply does not have the strength to carry on.

The third lesson that I learned was compassion. It is expressing kindness, sympathy, concern, and consideration. She was the first person that I had ever known that was sick. In my family, people were either alive or dead. They would literally be here one day and gone the next. But, they never suffered with illness for a long period of time. I have learned that sometimes you have to be a shoulder to cry on. Other times, they may just need to vent. Once in a while, you need to give advice. And always, try to make them laugh.

Finally, when your best friend has lupus, treat them like you would a best friend that does not have lupus. I do not treat her a certain way because she has lupus. I treat her with love because that is how I feel toward her. Being flexible, supportive and compassionate toward your friends is a courtesy that should be extended to anyone that you call friend. I am a firm believer in treating people the way that you want to be treated. To have a good friend you have to be a good friend

CHAPTER 22

Perspective Highlight – A Husband's Perspective

By Mickey Caruana

My name is Mickey Caruana. Lupus came into my life under cover of a stunning beauty with a great singing voice. It was a couple of months into our friendship before I found out lupus was the reason she disappeared for a couple of days after we had been working together and hanging out. I thought it was just the heavy workload and early mornings in nursing school. The phone calls were not returned immediately and I think I had to work a night or two without her there. It was a job she had gotten me, so I certainly noticed when she was missing.

We met at karaoke, and she did not know it was my first time hosting a karaoke show, but she told a newly opened bar and grill they needed to hire me. I did not let her disappear like I think she wanted to. It seemed she would rather fade from the friendship that had started developing than admit she was sick. It was not like she was trying to hide it, just embarrassed, almost ashamed, that there were some days it was almost impossible for her, a vibrant looking 25 year old, to get out of bed. But, she had to do that because she had to get up for school at 5:45 a.m., then work at night. The part that I think was the worst for her was telling people, her friends, peers, that hanging out or doing things that required her precious and limited amounts of energy was not possible.

I did not let her off the hook that easy, to just get away with not calling back. It wasn't just because I could not believe she was turning down a chance to talk to and hang out with me, I wanted to know what was going on that she seemed to want to withdraw from several new friendships. I remember asking, "Well, what it is? What do you mean you don't feel well, are you sick?" Thinking at first it was just the flu, the way she was afraid to talk about it, I thought, maybe cancer? When she said lupus, I said " I have no idea what that is, I just know the root Lupine means wolf, so is it wolf disease, and what does that mean?" In my head, I thought well at least it is not cancer or HIV.

She explained a little to me about the fatigue that plagued her and the occasional flare ups, mainly from stressful situations. I was just starting to lead a home fellowship that was going through the Purpose Driven Life study. She had accepted the invitation to attend, and with her permission, we kept her in prayer and got to know more about her and her struggles with this disease. Our friendship grew and the group and I prayed her through a really stressful time of facing a disability hearing. The medical and credit card bills had really piled high in the first few years of diagnosis, after she was coming out of rehab for being run over by a truck when the lupus came out of the shadows. Learning about these traumatic events, although some teeth had to be pulled, helped understand the initial hesitancy to share and explain an overwhelming set of tragedies. It made it more understandable why the dark cave of aloneness might seem comfortable. It was through this study of the Purpose Driven Life together that I saw a girl who lupus would attack, but who would not surrender. She had goals and a determination to see them through, but lupus had other plans.

I started dating that girl with lupus after we had been friends for several months. I knew a lot more about her and a little about the disease, not much really yet, but enough to develop a bit of a plan in my mind. I just got to know this girl and who she was, and realized her character was much greater than the lupus she had. I saw her deal with the anguish of her goal of finishing nursing school (where she was a straight A student) being crushed by lupus. I saw her struggle through this and never give up. I found out this was not the first time her plans were drastically altered by this illness. I also saw it was not the first time she had changed her course.

I ended up marrying that girl, and I will share very honestly how I answered the questions from concerned people who said, "Really, you are going to marry someone who you know has a debilitating disease?" I could stand at the altar with the healthiest girl, a professional athlete

even, and on our way to the hotel from the reception, a slip
and fall or a driving accident could drastically change her
life. Just because someone marries a "healthy" person does
not mean that person won't face a health crisis in the
future.

I just felt that facing this known challenge together
with this woman I fell in love with was worth it. I did then,
and still do, believe and hope that one day lupus will not be
our daily concern. I do pray and hope for a total healing,
even though a doctor will tell you they do not heal lupus,
they just treat it. So, if they want to call it remission for 40
years that is fine with me. I reasoned with myself that it is
like driving in the rain. If you drive cautiously, with the
care and attention you should in those driving conditions,
you will be able to safely maneuver even when the road
turns. Potholes, sharp turns, and sudden stops are just that
if you remembered you are driving in the rain, and with
lupus I would say remember to always drive like it is
pouring. The problem is, I have forgotten this at times and
so has my wife. This desire to go fast and take on life, full
speed ahead, does not just go away because you get
diagnosed with something like lupus. There are days we
drive really slow with the hazards on. We know why, but
everyone else looks at us funny.

When we first started dating, her embarrassment and
shame with her limitations due to lupus made her always
want me to not bring it up, not tell people that the reason
we could not join them at the picnic was because she was
sick or too tired. I had come to understand why she wanted

to do this and so we usually did leave that out of why we could not join them. I do have to say that I think this backfired on us.

Some friends and family then started to come up with their own reasons why we missed so many events – whether they thought perhaps we were in an argument, or one of us did not care for the people we were going to be around · there was plenty of speculation. After we got married, lupus really made a big showing in our life. Her grandmother got sick while we were away on our honeymoon and we rushed back a little early. That next month was horrible as her grandmother got worse; she got very sick and then her grandmother passed. This caused lupus to spiral out of control as they were very close and the passing was a big blow. There were some incidents that came up when nothing but the truth would work, and people became much more aware of lupus. There were many days we could not leave the house without the wheelchair. That is, if she could leave at all and was not confined almost entirely or entirely to bed.

Some friends and family handled this with understanding. There are others though, (and some of you who are affected by lupus might know these types of people), who can never get past the thought that a young person who needs to take a nap during the day is just "lazy." Or, people who write you off because lupus has weakened you so much that taking work outside the home is not really possible.

Those times of being bedridden and needing to keep a bedpan in the bedroom (when you're in your thirties), well, they are horrible. Unfortunately, as I said, some friends and family do not seem to care because they just do not understand. These times were tough for my wife; they were tough for me. She dealt with the physical pain, but being there or trying to be there with someone who is hurting and bouncing up and down on prednisone and Plaquenil · wow · that is also a bumpy and difficult road.

The best part of living with lupus has been how clearly the miracles we have experienced stand out with such a dark background. To some, they are coincidence, to me they are "Godincidents," but I like calling them "miracles." We have not needed a wheelchair now in a few years, thank God. During that time we were given the news of a brain aneurysm found in a scan; we had to wait several months for it to be checked again to see if there was any change, and after waiting and much prayer and fear, it was miraculously gone. Some small TIA's have occurred· five in total · but thank God, none with any lasting damage. It is just miraculous some days that after an extremely rough week, where she cannot decide whether she would rather kill herself or kill me, we still talk and then go to bed snuggling.

One miracle that I have been able to witness is God taking a broken, hurting girl who had concluded that nursing was her goal, and direct her otherwise. I think she settled with that for some of the wrong reasons, not because it was her gift and God's plan. Ah, but to watch when she does find herself discovering a gift she never really knew she had or ever thought to pursue, now that is something. To see doors open one at a time, starting small, doors she has to crawl through, but that prepare her for what is next. Then the miracle of getting fired because without that you would never have thought to take the next job that comes your way...a job that lets you learn and discover new things which you love to do and share that information in a story. Also, a job you can do from home, even from bed when necessary, and sometimes with a few naps in between. These are naps of exhaustion and fatigue from a constant fever for weeks that most healthy people would never try to or could not understand.

The miracle of perseverance, and the reward for the struggle – that is what I have been able to witness. Another door closed, another time of wondering why when it all seemed so good, such a fitting job taken away. Why? What now? Just as the body needs time to rest because Lupus is on the prowl. Then a door opens and it is an opportunity beyond expectation, but you realize had door number one not closed, door number two could not be entered. Then big change enters your life and along with it stress. Lights start flashing, "Watch out, Lupus is going to try and show up and steal this."

All of these things happened and I am so happy and proud to say that Marisa has met these challenges head on whether in bed with fever or standing strong. She now has a chance to share stories about what Lupus can do to a person, but more so that a person with Lupus can still do anything, and sometimes more than they ever dreamed.

My wife, that beautiful, karaoke singer I met, is Marisa... who as God would have it, is writing this book to help with lupus awareness and to help those with lupus know that lupus does not have to win.

My role in this? Marisa occasionally needs to be reminded on good days and bad, sometimes several times on good days and about two dozen times on bad days ,that even the prison of lupus has many escapes.

Highlighting and remembering miracles helps. Do not spend more time listing your symptoms and diagnosis than your blessings. Your symptoms will not change your life or the world, but how you react to them could. Really it could; even if that means it just changes one person's world, you are a world changer. Just learn to bite things off in sizes you can chew, so you don't choke on anything lupus throws your way. No one invites a constant choker to dinner, and driving badly in the rain is dangerous.

Remember when I said she would not surrender, but there were and are days of retreat, recouping, and regrouping, and sometimes just coasting? We had a lot of those over our first five years of marriage. Not now though, because there are times in life of doubling your efforts for a time to knock a couple of Lupus' teeth out. That time is now.

About the Author

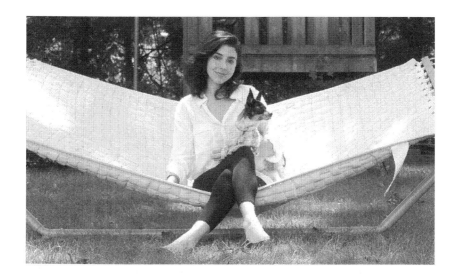

Marisa Zeppieri-Caruana is an author, freelance writer and speaker, currently residing in New York and Florida. Marisa has had over 300 articles published covering a wide variety of topics including health, business, religion, women's issues, and current events. She has been featured and interviewed on the topic of Lupus in *Glamour, Eating Well, WebMD, MSNBC, South Florida Today, The Good News, The Chicago Tribune* and *Yahoo*.

Formally educated in Chemistry and Fine Art, Marisa was about to graduate with her RN degree when she was diagnosed with Systemic Lupus. Confined to a bed, she rekindled her love for writing and embarked on a new and fulfilling career. She is currently working on her second Lupus related book and serves as a board member for the Lupus Foundation of America, Southeast Florida Chapter.

Marisa is also the founder of www.LupusSurvivalGuide.com, a website and blog designed for Lupus patients and their families, and www.Wordslingergal.com, a website for those interested in a writing career.

On her "good" Lupus days, Marisa enjoys cooking, spending time with her husband and rescue dog, working out via Xbox, and reading.

Acknowledgements

First, I thank God for not only giving me life, but also giving me a unique plan and purpose *for* my life. I pray this book brings glory to you, and encourages those who do not already know you to seek you out.

I thank both of my grandparents, Rosie and Bogey, for their never-ending support and unconditional love. Though you are both no longer here, I think about you daily. I thank you for providing one of the only stable homes I have known and for encouraging me, no matter what endeavor I was about to embark on.

Grandma, I am thankful for your crazed obsession with books. What I wouldn't give for one more trip to the library with you. My only regret is that I began my writing career after you passed. I dedicate every word I write to you. Bogey, I thank you for being an exceptional example of how a man should love and treat his family. Thank you for all of the arts and craft lessons, allowing me to shadow you in your woodshop, showing me how important it is to perform random acts of kindness, and for having such a loving and genuine heart.

A million thanks for my incredible mother. You are my rock, my friend, my encourager, my "pity party" attender and my "snap out of it already" enforcer. I am truly the luckiest daughter alive to have a mother who is compassionate, intelligent and kind. Thank you for tending to me during my worst times and celebrating with me during my best times. Thank you for all of the sacrifices you made in order to give your children the best life possible. And, thank you for encouraging me to explore a relationship with God. Your unwavering faith has helped to change both of our lives. You will always be my inspiration.

For my lovebug and very best friend, Mickey Caruana. Thanks for being a supportive husband and keeping me on course with this book, even when I was ready to put the project on the shelf. Thank you for the continuing encouragement that this book would be a reality one day. You are an incredibly patient soul to deal with a wife who has a chronic disease, is extremely Type A, and can be slightly annoying at times. I am blessed that you chose me to spend the rest of your life with and I am looking forward to many more happy and healthy years with one another. I cannot possibly tell you how thankful I am for you in one paragraph, but I believe this will say it all... *Yer jalan atthirari anni, Shekh ma shieraki anni.*

A gigantic hug to my best buds, Alan Pokotilow and Karla McLaren. What is better than having two friends who you can trust with your deepest secrets, laugh with until you can't breathe, and express yourself completely in front of, knowing you will never be judged? There is *nothing* better than having you two as my best friends. Alan, thanks for bringing silly board games to the hospital in order to lift my spirits, helping me play pranks on my grandmother, and introducing me to Matzo ball soup and black & white cookies. Karla, thank you for being a trustworthy, compassionate and kindhearted friend. Thank you for always having me in stitches, being my morning "coffee" phone call buddy, showing me how to really clean a kitchen (fast!), and being an incredible example of a faithful Christian woman.

Thank you to my older brother, Peter (PJ) Zeppieri, his amazing wife, Noelle, and new baby, Alexander. PJ, thank you for always offering help whenever I am in need, being a solid, dependable family member, and helping me and mom through some difficult times. Noelle, you are like a sister to me and I trust you with my life. I love the fact that you just "get" me (and vice versa). And, to handsome baby Alexander, I can't wait to spend more time with you and watch you grow up! You always put a smile on my face.

To Petagaye, thank you for being one of my dearest friends. I am grateful that we can pick up the phone at any time and continue exactly where we left off.

Thank you to the incredible men and women who shared their stories and helped make this book possible: Naomi Jeanty, Tanique Rose, Laurie Renfro, Damian Velez, Kim Green, Kia Paynes-Gentry, Patricia Guidice, Jessica Goldman Foung, Jody Ortiz, Kim Green, PJ Nunn, Nicole Francis, Linda Bernal Apgar, Kathleen Walker, Wendy Phillips, Elijah Julian Samaroo, and Jonathan Ramirez.

Thank you to Amy Kelly Yalden, CEO of the Lupus Foundation of America Southeast Florida Chapter, and Dr. Cadet for being integral parts of this book. Having you both share your knowledge and personal experiences with this disease were vital to the purpose and mission of this book. I believe this information is going to help many patients and their loved ones.

Other people who have made an impact in my life and have helped me either with this book or keep my sanity with this disease include Peter Zeppieri (Sr.), The Caruana family, William McLaren, Angela Zeppieri ,Troy Ansted, Erika Kay, Tricia Heng, Dr. Christian, Dr. Romero, Dr. Forstot, Dr. Dennis and Dr. Norberg.

Thank you to Thai Racer of www.Lifeionizers.com for your compassionate heart and reaching out to me to help with this disease. Your gift is proof that good people still exist in this world, and sometimes a helping hand will come from a complete stranger.

Also, many thanks to publicist PJ Nunn, (www.breakthroughpromotions.net), for sharing a wealth of knowledge regarding publicity and publishing.

Thanks to Mike Wall of Rockin' Wellness for creating a product that actually works...and tastes great! Also, for sharing your knowledge about the product and how it can help in my particular situation.

A special thank you to Stevan Jovanovic for a beautiful ebook cover.

I apologize in advance for anyone I may have left out. So many incredible people in my life have played a role in this book or have helped me immensely in dealing with this disease. For *all* of my friends and family, I thank you from the bottom of my heart.

In Memory Of...

This book is in memory of Erin Kelly. Erin, although I never met you, I know you would be so proud of everything your sister, Amy, is doing for lupus patients and how she is using your story to educate others. She is truly incredible and I am thankful God has blessed me with her friendship.

Made in the USA
San Bernardino, CA
03 September 2016